Environmental Factors Affecting Human Health

Edited by Ivan Uher

Published in London, United Kingdom

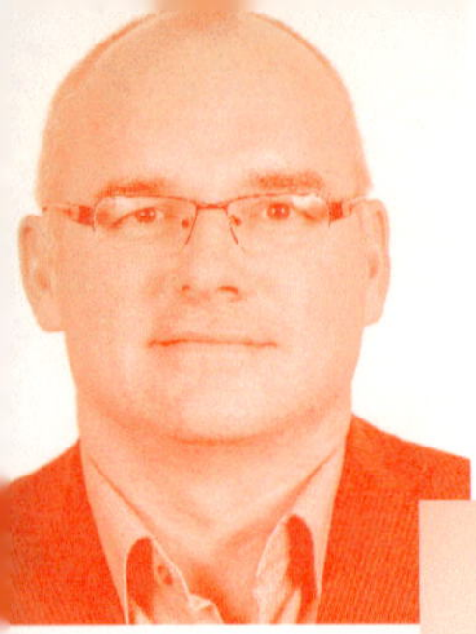
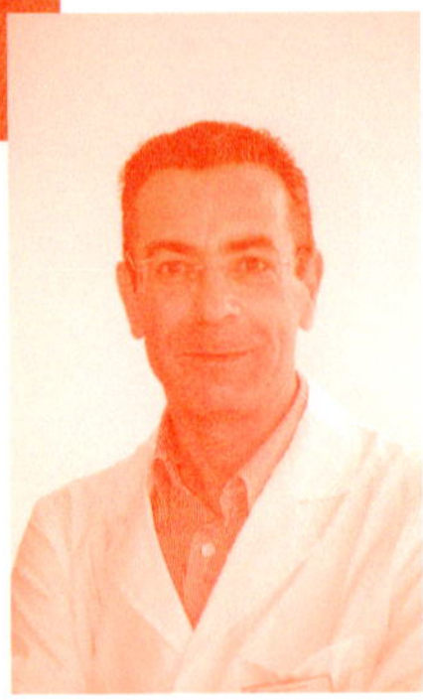
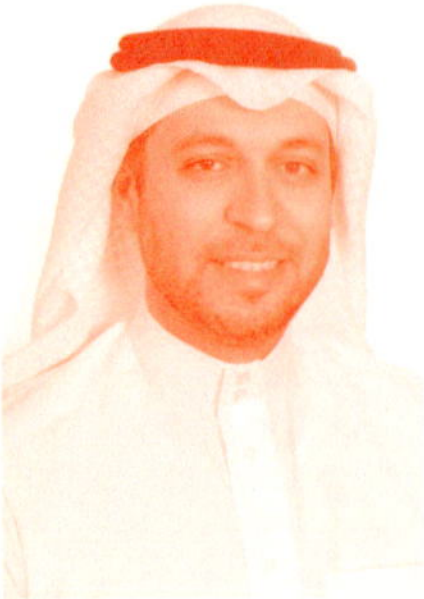
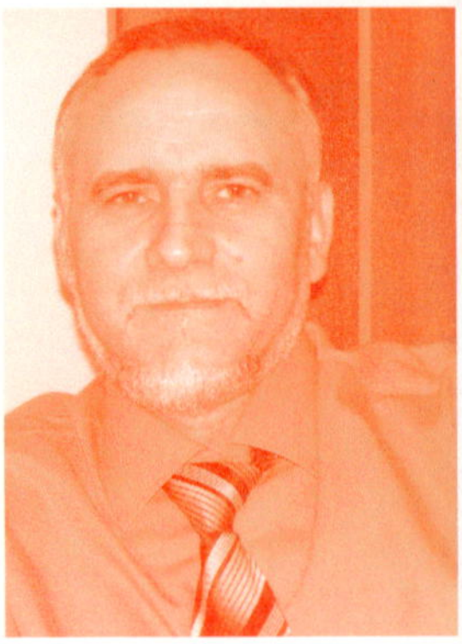
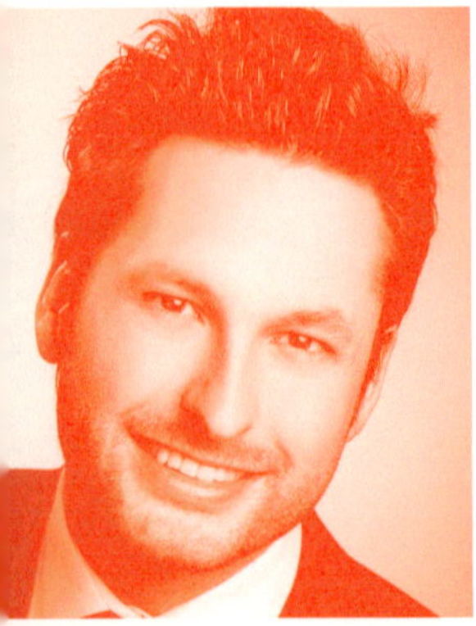
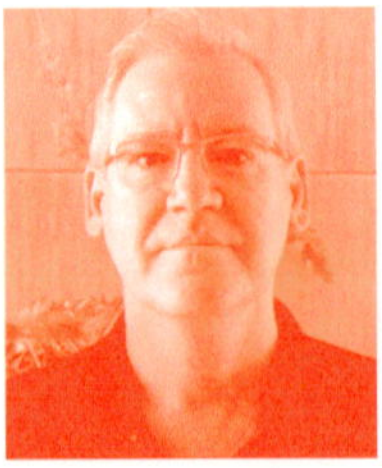
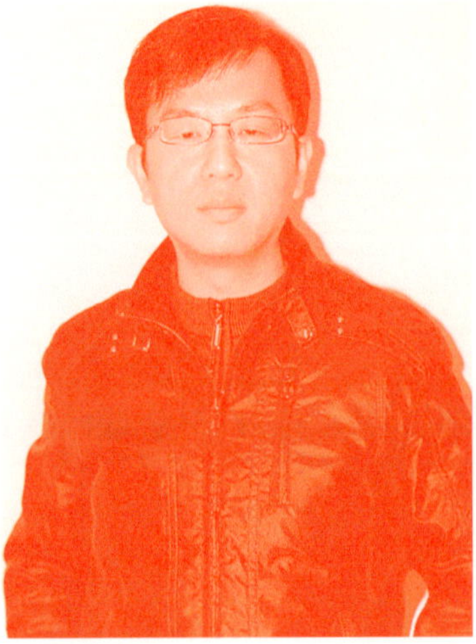

IntechOpen

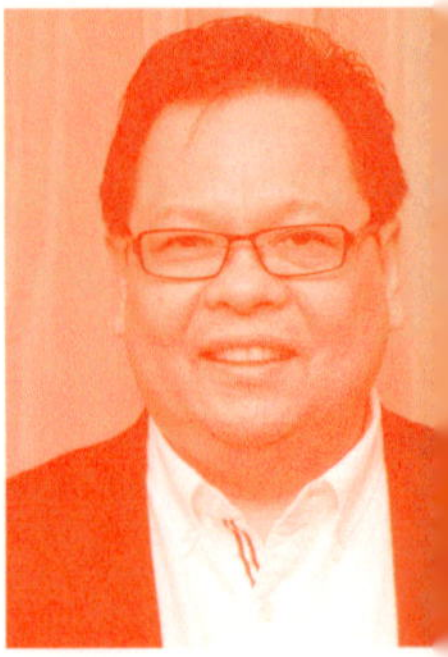
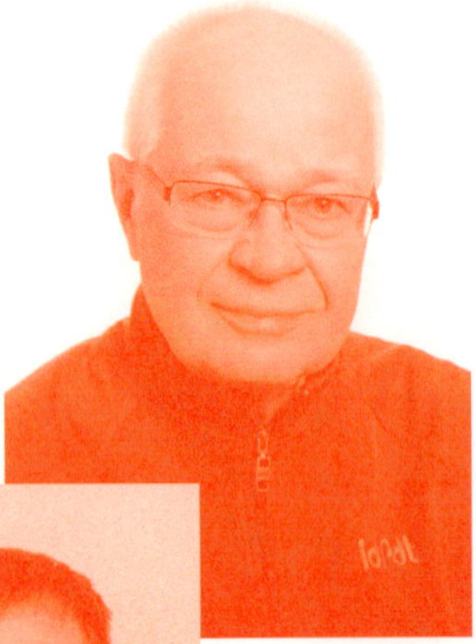
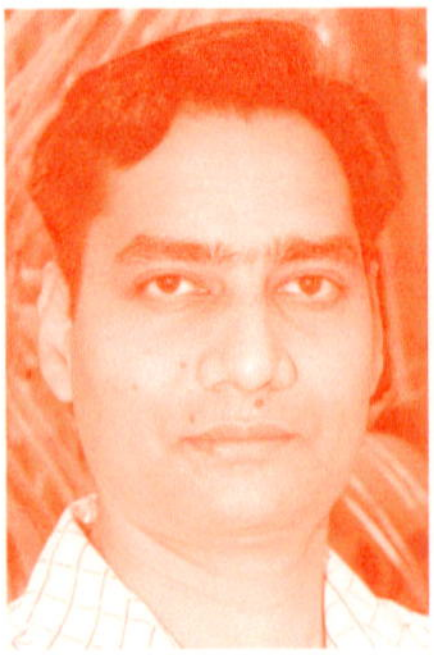
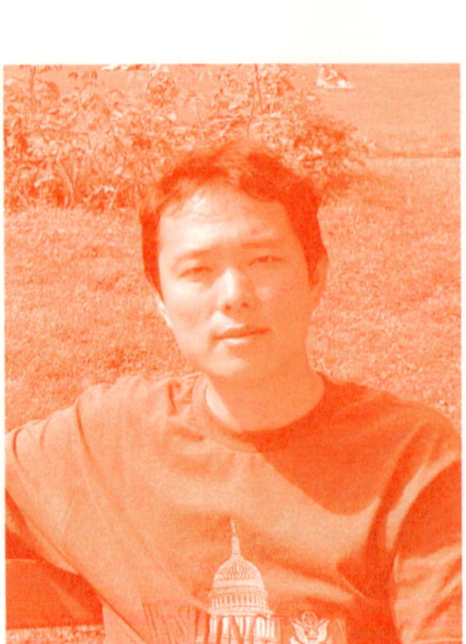
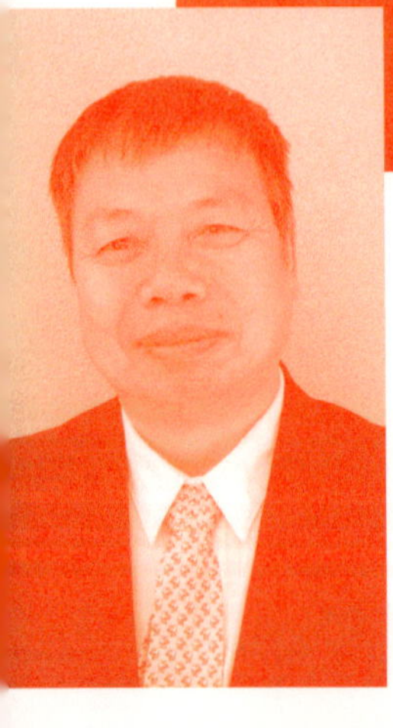
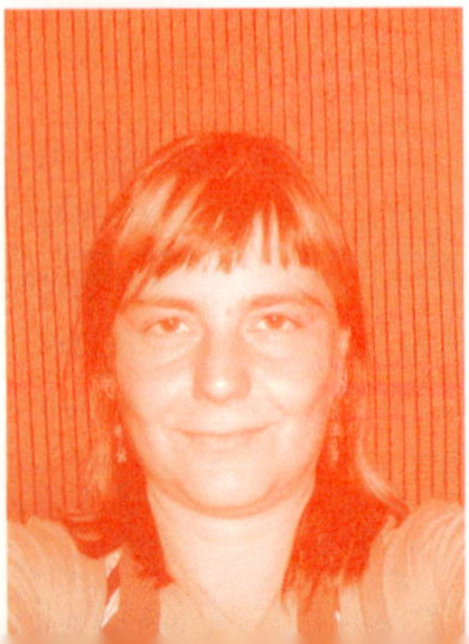

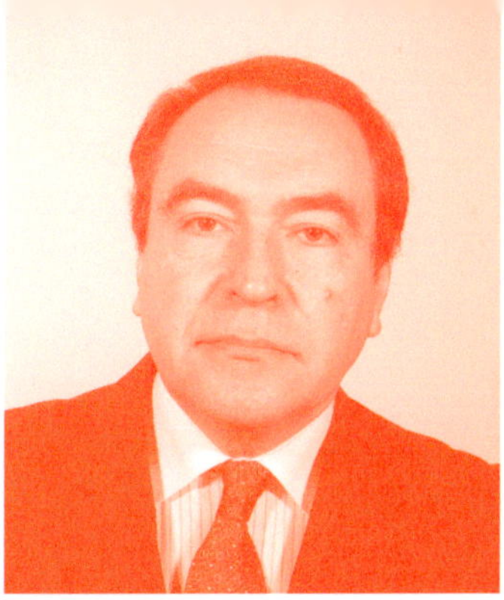
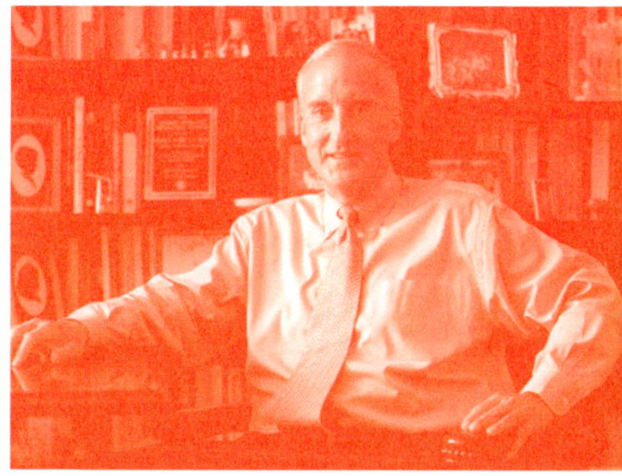
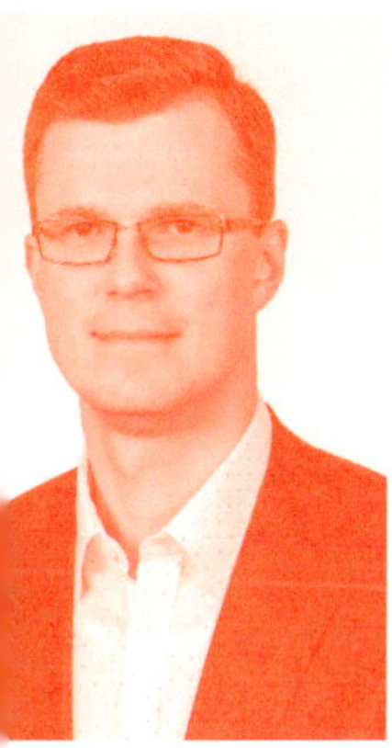
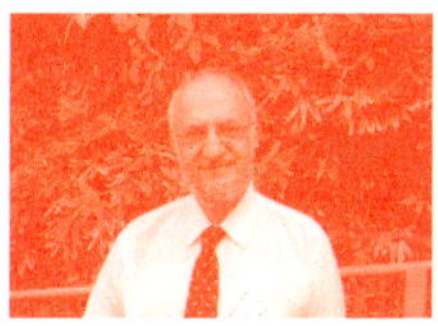
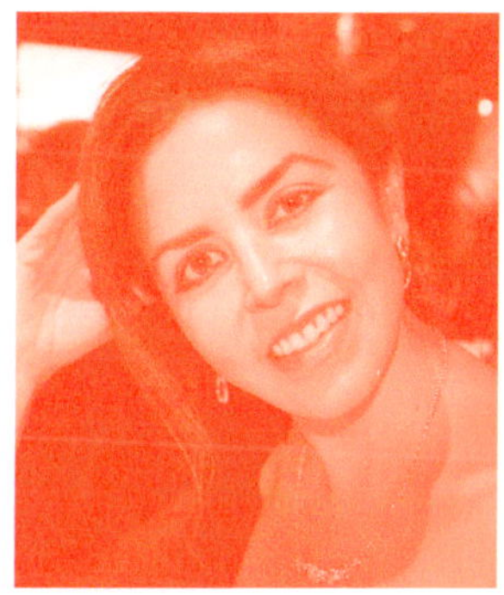

Supporting open minds since 2005

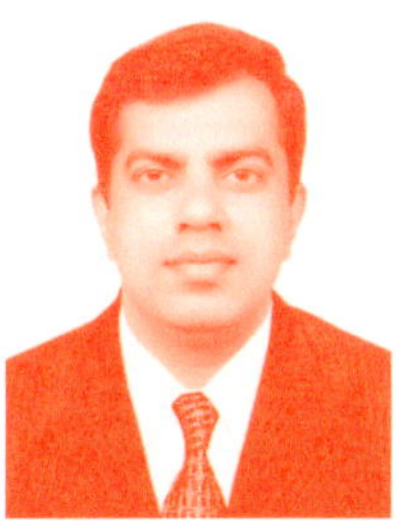
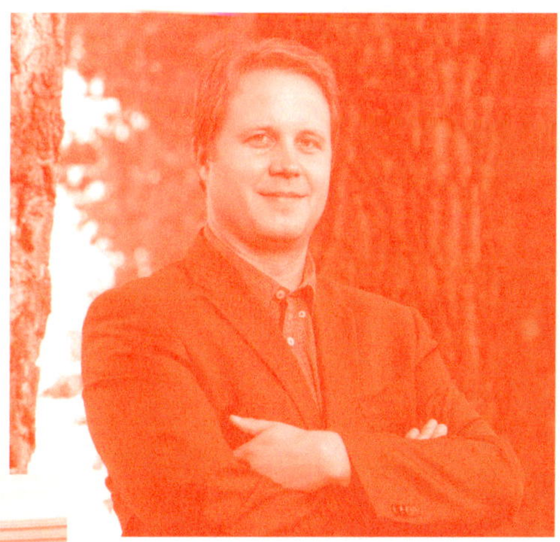
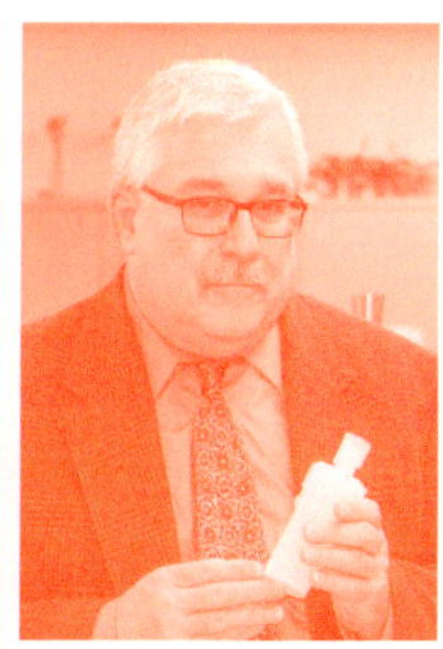
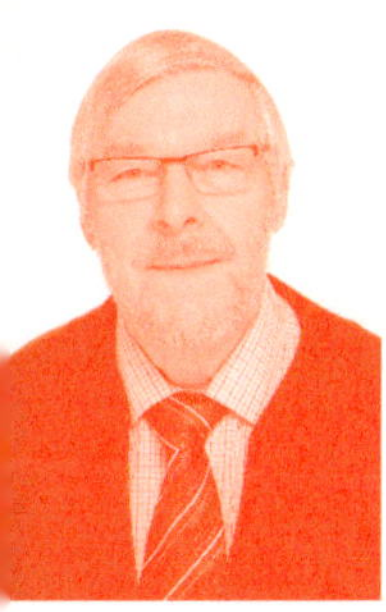
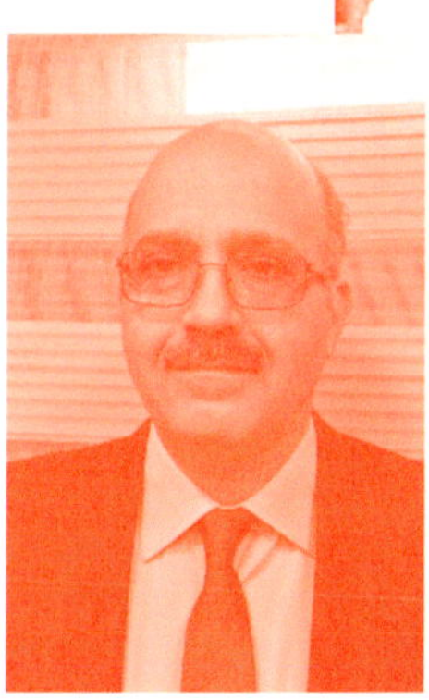
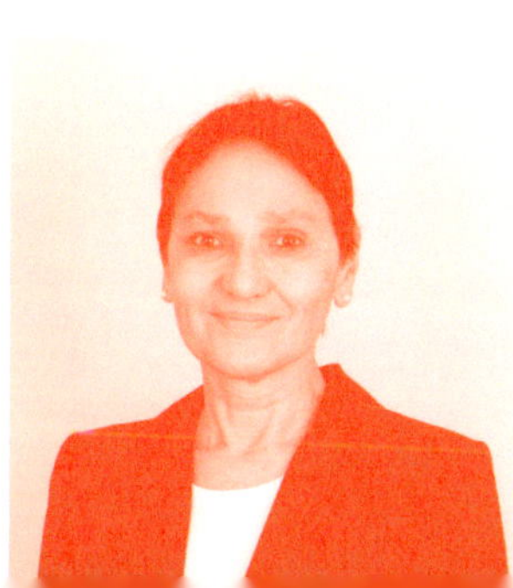
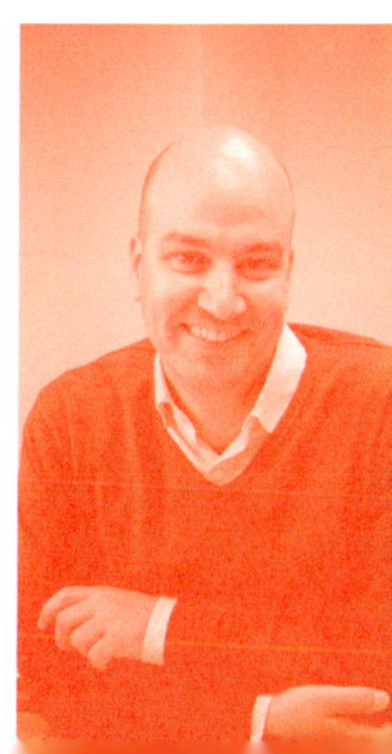

Environmental Factors Affecting Human Health
http://dx.doi.org/10.5772/intechopen.81138
Edited by Ivan Uher

Contributors
Gun Mardiatmoko, Jan Willem Hatulesila, Andrés Ursa Herguedas, Femi Ilevbare, Takemi Otsuki, John Kanayochukwu Nduka, Henriette Ijeoma Kelle, Iveta Cimboláková, Ivan Uher, Katarína Veszelits Laktičová, Mária Vargová, Tatiana Kimáková, Ingrid Papajová, Peter Korim, Rudolf Hromada, Emre Babur, A. Krishnaveni, M. Pandiyan Muthaiyan, Sivakumar Chinnasamy, Jamuna Elumalai, Naoko Kumagai-Takei, Suni Lee, Kei Yoshitome, Nagisa Sada, Yasumitsu Nishimura, Turgay Dindaroglu, Emeka Chima Ogoko, Perpetua Chioma Okafor

First published in London, United Kingdom, 2020 by IntechOpen
IntechOpen is the global imprint of INTECHOPEN LIMITED, registered in England and Wales, registration number: 11086078, 7th floor, 10 Lower Thames Street, London, EC3R 6AF, United Kingdom
Printed in Croatia

British Library Cataloguing-in-Publication Data
A catalogue record for this book is available from the British Library

Additional hard and PDF copies can be obtained from orders@intechopen.com

Environmental Factors Affecting Human Health
Edited by Ivan Uher
p. cm.
Print ISBN 978-1-78985-527-2
Online ISBN 978-1-78985-528-9
eBook (PDF) ISBN 978-1-83962-853-5

For EU product safety concerns:
IN TECH d.o.o., Prolaz Marije Krucifikse Kozulić 3, 51000 Rijeka, Croatia, info@intechopen.com or visit our website at intechopen.com.

Meet the editor

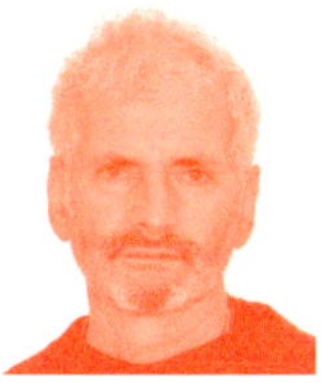

Dr. Ivan Uher is working as an Associate Professor at Pavol Jozef Šafarik University, Slovakia. His research includes the following fields: aging, physiology in sport and exercise, health and nutrition, lifestyle in prevention and treatment of health problems, and quality of life. He has more than 100 publications in scientific journals and books and has held lectures, seminars, and workshops in various conferences.

Contents

Preface

We often fail to acknowledge that knowledge is multiplicative, and technologies are synergistic. Humankind is far more innovative than we give it credit. Over the past hundred years, generation after generation has witnessed the appearance of innovative technologies. At first, we were shocked, and then we barely notice the global changes in our environment. Advances in the field of environmental health taught us much about human health hazards. In that respect, environmental health and the natural environment requires us to redefine our approach, at the same time readiness to engage in a multiplicity of approaches.

The present book examines the issues of potential risk (e.g., environmental contaminants, climate, and seasonal changes benefits of decomposition process on the soil also discussing collective defense, universal vulnerability, and global responsibility that can build a safer future for the humanity). We intended to present thoughts, processes, and techniques to convey environmental risks and susceptibility, make public the comprehensive interactions between nature and human pursuits.

The first two chapters evaluate global challenges of climate change in the Eastern region of Indonesia and Nigeria. Particularly its health risks, discomfort for urban and rural communities, emphasizing governmental responsibility to raise awareness, following necessary steps, especially for the most vulnerable social groups. The third and the forth chapters deal with environmental contaminants that play a crucial role in the transmission of pathogens. The chapters examine the structure of sanitation (i.e., methods, stages of disinfection, environmental factors) that influence the effectiveness of disinfection, addressing nonmonotonic dose-response relationships (hormesis). Also, the authors attempted to quantify the relationship between exposure of heavy metals on the organism via the atmosphere, hydrosphere, and pedosphere.

The fifth chapter looks into specific environmental substances such as asbestos fibers and silica particles that yield various health issues. This chapter summarizes the effect of those substances on the human immune system and outlines future direction in the research and practice. The sixth chapter emphasizes a holistic approach to the most common health issues of our civilization.

They were focusing on collective defense, universal vulnerability, and global solidarity, where the international public health action can build a safer future for humanity. The seventh chapter looks into seasonal changes of soil microbial biomass, and soil organic carbon in the karst ecosystem. The author of this chapter presents the most important factors of soil quality and health factors managing soil carbon in forest soils and provides us with how seasonal changes affect soil organic carbon and microbial biomass carbon. The eighth chapter describes sugar industry wastes as an organic plant material that returns to the soil and, through the decomposition process, provides nutrients and habitat to organisms living in the soil and, at the same time, binds soil particles and improves the water holding capacity of the soil. The last chapter looks into the impact of automobile and automobile transportation and its detrimental effect on the environment and public health in Nigeria.

Despite all the negative impacts on the environment, we have to be aware that a fresh wave of technological innovation is amplifying our understanding of complex environmental challenges and thus giving us new means to solve them. New technologies should help us (countries, companies, and citizens) to see problems, identify opportunities, and measure progress; proving that technology can help us save the planet. But more than anything, we must learn to value our nature. On this road we have to change how we grow, buy and choose what to eat. The fundamental question is whether new technologies have the potential to shift the current model to a more advanced system that could leave producers, consumers, and the planet better off. Ultimately, the positive changes in our lifestyle will benefit not only the individual, but also the community, society in which we live, our near and distant environment, and therefore the planet as a whole.

Dr. Ivan Uher
Pavol Jozef Šafárik University,
Košice, Slovakia

Chapter 1

Effects of Climate Change on City Life: Case Study in the City of Ambon, Indonesia East Region

Gun Mardiatmoko and Jan Wilem Hatulesila

Abstract

It is no stranger that the diminishing amount of forest land to become non-forested in the world has changed the microclimate in almost all urban and rural areas. Thus it globally has triggered climate change. The influence of forests or vegetated areas on climate, especially the microclimate and mesoclimate, is important. The disrupted microclimate will cause anomalies in elements of the microclimate such as rainfall, air temperature, relative humidity, solar radiation, wind, etc. Microclimate changes will affect the presence of forests in the region because plants have a large dependence on climate and weather conditions. The impact of climate change that is beginning to be seen and felt today has caused discomfort for urban and rural communities. The aim of this present paper is to investigate the comfort level of the population and the availability of green open space (GOS) in Ambon City, Maluku Province, Indonesia. The city of Ambon turned out to provide less comfort for residents who live there. Extreme rainfall has triggered the occurrence of flooding and has been detrimental to city residents, especially during the rainy season. On the contrary, very hot weather in the dry season has made city residents uncomfortable. This situation was triggered by the expansion of settlement construction in protected forest areas as a result of humanitarian riots that occurred in years 1999–2002, limited GOS, and the effects of climate change.

Keywords: extreme rainfall, flooding, microclimate, green open spaces, NDVI, GIS

1. Introduction

It is no stranger that forest areas and other vegetation areas are balancing components of various cycles in nature, including for circulation of climate and local-scale weather. Utomo argues that climate is a generalization of various weather conditions in a large area in a long time. Climates always change according to space and time. Based on certain timescale, climate change will form a particular pattern or cycle, daily, seasonal, annual, and several yearly cycles [1]. In addition to changes in patterned cycles, human activity causes climate patterns to change sustainably, both on a global and local scale. Forests regulate the temperature of the earth and weather patterns which are carried out by storing large amounts of carbon and water. This function as regulator also has a huge influence on the local climate. The role of forests as a regulator of the microclimate in the surrounding environment is very important [2]. Of course the different conditions of the forest in an area have different capabilities in regulating the microclimate in the forest environment, for example, air temperature, air humidity, reception of sunlight, and deficit of water vapor pressure. In general, the microclimate that arises is caused by the existence of various differences from the weather and climate conditions which are quite large, especially the physical properties of the atmosphere. Air temperature near the surface of the ground is strongly influenced by the amount of solar radiation absorbed by the surface of the soil itself. Some of the radiation received by the soil surface during the day is used to heat and propagate to deeper parts, and some of it is irradiated in the form of heat waves that heat the air and evaporate water. Short energy solar radiation that propagates into the soil is converted into heat energy in the soil which will affect the temperature of the soil.

The influence of forests on climate is very important with increasing forest area and forest stand density. At first the forest compiler vegetation was only affected by microclimate, but later it was gradually influenced by the macroclimate and mesoclimate. Climate elements that affect the growth of vegetation include rainfall, temperature, wind, sunlight, humidity, and evapotranspiration. In other words there is a close relationship between climate patterns and the distribution of forest stands. Therefore some climate classifications are based on the world of vegetation. Vegetation has been seen as something sensitive and complex to climate influences, such as solar radiation, heating of soil and air, soil and air humidity, and so on. Seeing the close relationship between forests and climate, the increasing number of forest areas that have been converted into non-forest areas resulting in degradation and deforestation in almost all parts of the world has triggered climate change. The impact of this climate change has caused human misery both in urban and rural areas. This paper intends to describe a city whose population is uncomfortable due to the many natural disasters that occur because of the illegal settlements of protected forest areas in the center of Ambon Island. Besides that, it is also due to the limited GOS in the city. This happened because of conflicts in the nuances of the tribe, religion, and race (TRR) that occurred in years 1999–2002.

2. Methodology

This research uses survey and descriptive methods. The study was conducted in Ambon City, Maluku Province, Indonesia. Ambon City or Ambonese is a big city and also the capital of Maluku Province with a land area of 359.45 km^2 and a sea area of 17.55 km^2 with a coastline length of 98 Km. At present, "Ambon Manise" has become a more advanced city and is regarded as an international city in Eastern Indonesia. The administrative area of Ambon City is 377 km^2 or 2/5 of the area of Ambon Island. Geographically, Ambon City is located 3° 34' 8.40 "–3° 47' 42.00" south latitude and 128° 1′ 33.60 "–128° 18' 3.60" east longitude. Geographically, this city on Ambon Island is surrounded by the sea. This causes Ambon City to have two seasons, namely, tropical climate and seasonal climate. The location of Ambon City is bordered by the Banda Sea on the south, the Central Maluku Regency on the east (Lease Islands), the land of Hila-Leihitu and Kaitetu-Leihitu on the west, and Salahutu District, Central Maluku, on the north. At present, Ambon City is divided into five sub-districts, Nusaniwe, Sirimau, Teluk Ambon, Teluk Baguala, and Leitimur Selatan, which are divided into 50 villages. The area of the study covers three administrative villages, namely, Honipopu Village, Ahusen Village, and Uritetu Village, with an area of 1,115,900 m^2 or 111.6 ha. This location is the entire GOS area of the Ambon City.

To find out rainfall patterns and climate information in Ambon City, it was conducted by collecting various climate data, i.e., humidity, precipitation, wind, temperature, etc., and the history of natural disasters in Ambon City. Based on everyday experience, if we are in a vegetated area, it will feel cooler and more comfortable. This is especially felt during the daytime during the dry season. This is closely related to air humidity and air temperature conditions around us. In this regard, to analyze the distribution of humidity, air temperature, and its relation to a fairly extensive urban vegetation distribution, spatial analysis on the geographical information system (GIS) can be used. Besides that, the normalized difference vegetation index (NDVI) approach is also used to monitor vegetated areas. NDVI quantifies vegetation by measuring the difference between near-infrared (NIR) (which vegetation strongly reflects) and red light (which vegetation absorbs) [3]. Remote sensing and GIS technology have advanced rapidly in recent decades and now play an important role in environmental fields, i.e., climate science, biodiversity conservation, forestry, urban–rural planning, land and water management, etc. Thus spatial data is becoming increasingly accessible and used by various governments and research institutions, private businesses, consulting companies, and others.

The distribution of vegetation in Ambon City is obtained by the NDVI value approach. The vegetation index value is calculated as the measured reflection ratio of the red (R) and near-infrared (NIR) bands on the electromagnetic wave spectrum. Both of these bands were chosen as vegetation index parameters because the measurement results were most affected by the absorption of leaf chlorophyll or green vegetation. In general the NDVI formula is written with the following equation:

$$\mathrm{NDVI} = (\mathrm{NIR} - \mathrm{R})/(\mathrm{NIR} + \mathrm{R}) \tag{1}$$

where NIR is near-infrared and R is infrared. NDVI is classified into four classes of greenness level as presented in **Table 1**.

Through the NDVI distribution map, a ground check was then carried out. Locations selected, for example, are determined considering places that have high, medium, and low NDVI values and are not vegetated. In this case, nine sample points are set to take observational data in the field which include the distribution of vegetation (grass and trees), air temperature, air humidity, solar radiation, and noise that are evenly distributed in urban areas. The location mapping activity was carried out directly on the green lane along the road and the city park area in the corner of Ambon City spatial planning, and the distribution of the stand inventory lane was adjusted to the potential of plant species to facilitate recording and measurement. Vegetation mapping in open green areas in the spatial layout is done by GIS using ArcGIS 10.1 software. The collection of vegetation (grass and trees) plot points is carried out using global positioning system (GPS). Landsat ETM-8 imagery is processed using ENVI 4.7 and MAPINFO 10.5 software for merging image data bands. To find out the value of DI in this study, use the formula of DI [5] as follows:

$$\mathrm{DI} = \mathrm{Ta}–\mathbf{0.55}\ (\mathbf{1}–\mathbf{0.01}\ \mathrm{RH})\ (\mathrm{Ta}–\mathbf{14.5}) \tag{2}$$

where **DI** is the value of discomfort index, **Ta** is the air temperature, and **RH** is the relative humidity (%). DI is classified into six discomfort classes as presented in **Table 2**.

Based on the discomfort value in **Table 2**, three discomfort distribution maps are made, each of which includes six discomfort classes for Ambon city at 09:00–12:00 pm and 16:00 pm. Ground check is carried out in nine sampling locations by observing the discomfort distribution map created. The interview activities were carried out to 150 respondents or 150 head of families aged between 30 and 60 years at the sampling location. The aim is to see representation in capturing

No.	Vegetation index class	Greeness level
1	0.40–1	High
2	0.25–< 0.40	Medium
3	0.03–< 0.25	Low
4	−1–< 0.03	Non-vegetated

Source: Marwoto and Ginting [4].

Table 1.
Vegetation index class (NDVI).

No.	Discomfort index	Discomfort condition	Remarks
1.	DI < 21	Comfort	100% comfortable
2.	22 ≤ DI ≤ 24	Less than 50% of the population feel discomfortable	50% uncomfortable
3.	25 ≤ DI ≤ 27	More than 50% of the population feel discomfortable	60% uncomfortable
4.	27 ≤ DI ≤ 29	Most of the population feel discomfortable	70% uncomfortable
5.	30 ≤ DI ≤ 32	High-level discomfort	80% uncomfortable
6.	DI ≥ 32	Need health services	100% uncomfortable

Table 2.
Classification of discomfort index *value [4].*

information and data on population comfort levels related to the existence of GOS in Ambon City. The next step is to overlay the NDVI distribution map with the three discomfort distribution maps. Thus three new maps were obtained, i.e., the NDVI distribution index map and discomfort in Ambon City at 09:00–12:00 pm and 16:00 pm.

3. Results and discussion

3.1 Rainfall and extreme distribution of rainfall and flooding in Ambon City

The climate in Ambon City is classified as a tropical climate with significant rainfall with precipitation even during the driest month. The climate here is classified as Af based on the Köppen-Geiger system. The average rainfall is 3392 mm, and the average temperature in Ambon City reaches 26.5°C. The lowest average precipitation in November is 103 mm, while the highest is 622 mm in June (**Figure 1**).

In connection with the highest precipitation, the months June, July, and August are the months of caution for the city government and residents of Ambon City because it is the time of natural disasters (floods and landslides). The average air temperature is 27.5°C in January which is the hottest month and 25.0°C in July which is the coldest month of the year (**Figure 2**).

Between the driest and wettest months, the difference in precipitation is 519 mm. The variation in annual temperature is around 2.5°C. The Ambon City climate is presented in **Table 3.**

During the last 7 years, there have been at least four floods, i.e., in year 2012, 2013, 2016, and 2017. Floods occurred in August 2012 in inundated five subdistricts: Nusaniwe, Sirimau, Ambon Bay, Baguala, and Leitimur [7]. In the village

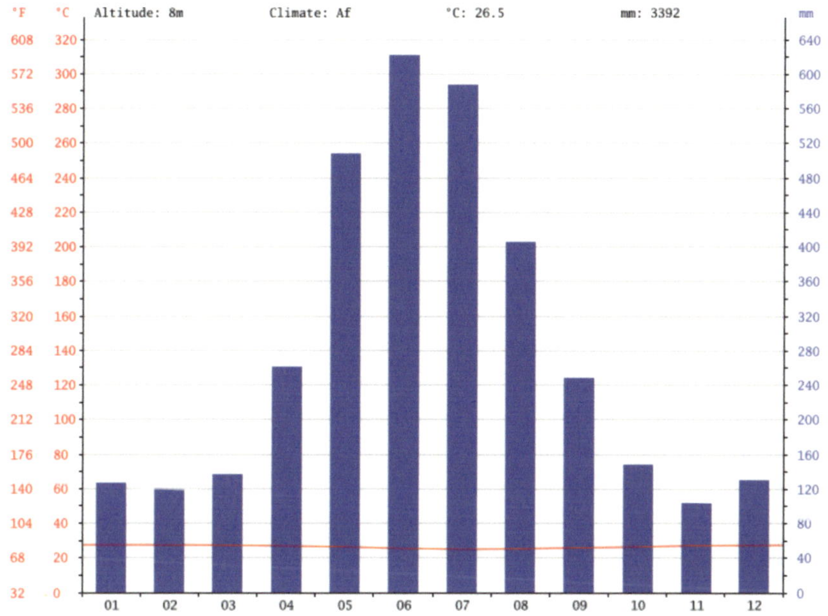

Figure 1.
Ambon City climate. Source: Climate-Data [6].

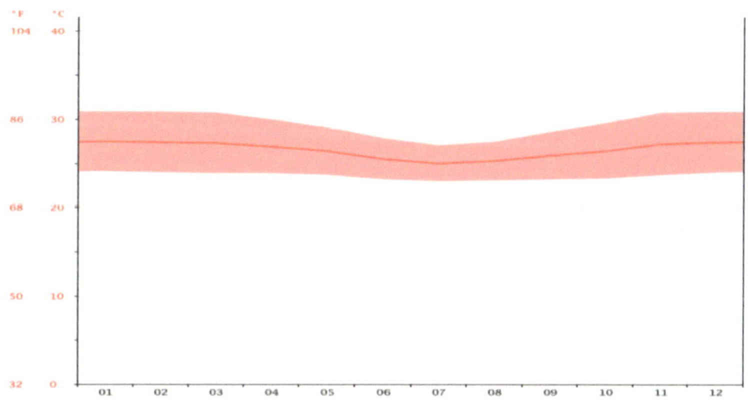

Figure 2.
Air temperature of Ambon City. Source: Climate-Data [6].

of Galala, floods soaked dozens of homes with 50 cm of water. In addition, the 3-m-high river water barrier and sea waves beside the Galala Bridge were damaged and collapsed [8]. Floods in year 2013 also occurred due to heavy rain for 2 days, July 29–30, 2013 [9]. These massive floods and landslides have caused 14 fatalities and forced thousands of residents to leave their homes and left huge infrastructure and environmental damage. The natural floods and landslides occurred again on July 16–17 and July 29–August 1, 2016. This disaster has caused damage to infrastructure and public facilities so that it covers the street body and shoulders at 10 points [10]. Moreover, floods also occur in the following year, 2017. A little description of the rainfall situation that triggers the occurrence of flooding is as follows: the rainfall in the Maluku Province exceeds the normal limit in the period of June 1–14, 2017. The amount of rainfall then continues to increase because it is the peak month of rain. Based on the Council of Meteorology, Climatology, and Geophysics measurements recorded 842 mm while normal rainfall in June ranges

	Jan	Feb	Mar	Apr	May	Jun	Jul	Aug	Sep	Oct	Nov	Dec
Average temperature (°C)	27.5	27.4	27.3	26.9	26.4	25.5	25	25.3	25.9	26.4	27.2	27.4
Minimum temperature (°C)	24.1	24	23.9	23.9	23.7	23.2	23	23.1	23.2	23.3	23.7	24
Maximum temperature (°C)	30.9	30.9	30.8	30	29.1	27.9	27.1	27.5	28.6	29.6	30.8	30.9
Average temperature (°F)	81.5	81.3	81.1	80.4	79.5	77.9	77.0	77.5	78.6	79.5	81.0	81.3
Minimum temperature (°F)	75.4	75.2	75.0	75.0	74.7	73.8	73.4	73.6	73.8	73.9	74.7	75.2
Maximum temperature (°F)	87.6	87.6	87.4	86.0	84.4	82.2	80.8	81.5	83.5	85.3	87.4	87.6
Precipitation/rainfall (mm)	126	118	136	261	508	622	587	405	248	148	103	130

Source: Climate-Data [6].

Table 3.
Weather by month/weather averages of Ambon City.

from 690 mm. This increase actually happened in the previous month (May 2017) where it was recorded at the Pattimura Ambon Meteorological Station, which was 753.3 mm, significantly exceeding normal rainfall of 400–500 mm. In addition the wind speed reaches 10–40 km/hour where the wind blows from east to southeast. This high rainfall is generally due to closed circulation around the Makassar Strait, attracting most of the saturated mass from the southern Pacific region through a large portion, Maluku region. As a result, there is a change in air mass in the central and northern Maluku regions. Meanwhile, the air humidity of the upper layers of the Maluku region shows a relatively wet condition (80–100%), which indicates the addition of water vapor supply. This is what drives the occurrence of high rainfall which will result in floods and landslides [11]. As a result of the overflowing of a number of rivers in the city of Ambon, dozens of houses and some roads in the city were submerged.

The amount of damage caused by floods is triggered by extreme rainfall, and there are also violations of the stipulated city spatial plan. As is known, Ambon City had been hit by social unrest motivated by the TRR between years 1999 and 2002. Residents of Ambon City felt the bad effects of riots that occurred more than a decade ago. One prominent factor is the construction of settlements that violate many spatial rules that have been set by the Ambon City government such as land clearing for settlements, agriculture and other activities in protected forests, etc. After the year of TRR conflict, many new settlements were built very heavily on cliffs, riverbanks, and valleys that were very risky for natural disasters. The most severe is the expansion of settlements in protected forest areas of Gunung Sirimau. This condition is exacerbated by the behavior of people who carelessly dispose of and accumulate garbage in places and areas that are not supposed to. This has an impact on natural disasters that are increasingly common in Ambon City and Islands. Ambon Island as a whole has a high disaster risk index.

In connection with the more frequent occurrence of floods, the Maluku Regional Development Planning Agency (BAPPEDA) has made the map of flood risk of Ambon City. The map was made from data on capacity and vulnerability of Ambon City to disaster and also disaster map of Ambon City (**Figure 3**). In this figure, it can be seen that almost half of Ambon City has a medium and high level of flood risk (yellow and red area).

Nara has analyzed rainfall trends toward extreme data on watersheds on Ambon Island for 32 years (1984–2015). In this study, the Mann-Kendall method and extreme value theory (EVT) were used to discuss extreme events that occurred and were modeled with the generalized extreme value (GEV) distribution, and the result was a trend of changes in rainfall in Ambon city. The annual maximum daily rainfall occurs in year 1984 which is 430.70 mm, and the minimum is 0 mm in year 1999, 2001, and 2003. Average rainfall varies between years 1984 and 2015, which is 25.63 to 131.408 mm, while the average value is 181.07 mm [13]. The distribution of average monthly rainfall in the study area tends to increase rainfall for 32 years but is not too significant because the rainfall data series is put together. Statistically, a significant trend was found for 8 months with an upward trend (positive) and 4 months experiencing a downward trend (negative). In other words, in a year there is an upward trend (positive) for 8 months, and the trend decreases for 4 months significantly (α = 0.05), and there is an increase in rainfall for the period of 1984–2015. Based on the results of the tests conducted, it has provided an analysis that rainfall data follows the form of GEV distribution with an average (μ) = 38,629, standard deviation (σ) = 36.64, and shape (ξ) = 0.436. This proves that rainfall in the watershed in Ambon Island has extreme distribution and has a maximum value distribution function for observing a period that is appropriate for the return period [13].

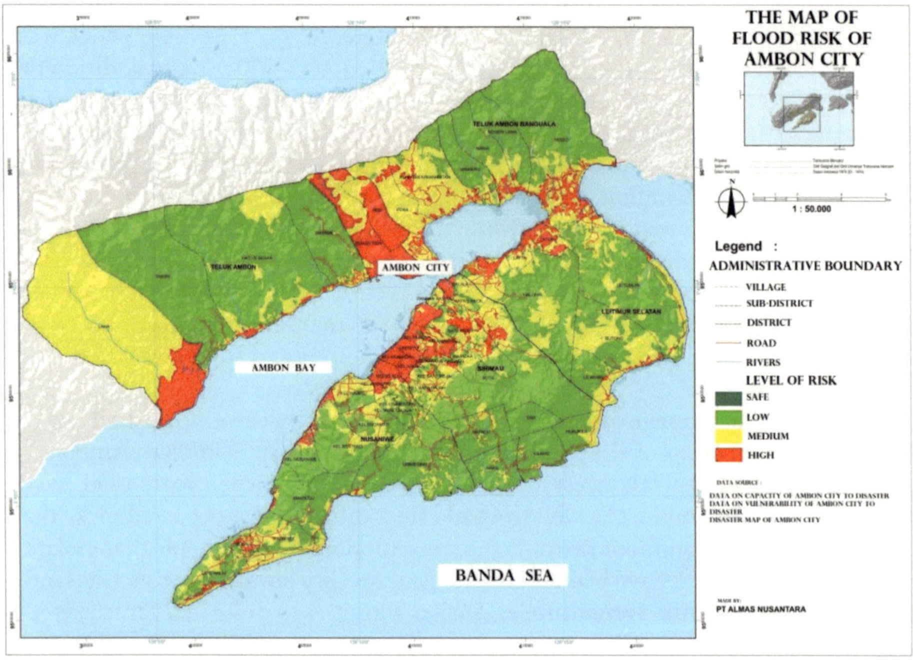

Figure 3.
The map of flood risk of Ambon City. Source: BAPPEDA Maluku [12].

3.2 Comfortability of city residents in Ambon City

The ideal climate for humans is clean air with temperatures of approximately 27–28°C and air humidity between 40 and 75% [14]. However, this condition often changes in a certain period of time which is quite drastic. This is caused by a significant change in land use, due to changes in the designation function, for example, from forested land to non-forest. Not only humans, in fact flora and fauna also often feel unfavorable effects due to changes in microclimate conditions, especially air temperature and air humidity [14]. If based on Laurie's opinion in 1986, the population of Ambon City is far from ideal climate conditions. Based on our direct measurement, results in 2017 are as follows: air temperature at 09:00, 12:00 pm, and 16:00 pm, respectively, is 26.73–29.97°C, 30.60–35.00°C, and 27.70–33.43°C; air humidity, respectively, is 85.67–97.00%, 35.00–64.33%, and 57.67%; and solar radiation, respectively, is 95–617 lux, 150–1299 lux, and 126–1252 lux. This situation will worsen if the wind speed on a certain day is very low. It is not surprising that the use of fans and air conditioners in government and private offices, shopping centers, and settlements has increased from year to year. Actually, this can be slightly overcome by the existence of urban green space (UGS)-GOS which is filled with a variety of vegetation. Unfortunately the existence of UGS-GOS is still very limited. UGS, green open space, city parks, vegetation areas, and others are useful in maintaining the natural balance of the city structure. Green spaces should not be considered as inefficient land or reserve land for urban development or simply a beauty program because they play a major role in balance, continuity, sustainability, comfort, health, and improvement of the quality of the city environment [15].

In general the development of urban areas will increase over time. The availability of facilities and infrastructure in urban areas to meet the living needs of the population (boards, food, clothing, vehicles, entertainment, etc.) has encouraged the increasing number of villagers to move toward urban areas or urbanization.

Of course cities that have exceeded their carrying capacity will have many negative impacts on the environment. Not infrequently if in a large city, there are certain areas that are not maintained, slum, dirty, and become a source of criminalization. Having created a peaceful atmosphere from the existence of a patterned conflict of TRR in years 1999–2002 has triggered massive urbanization which will negatively impact the comfort of living in Ambon City. Therefore, it is not surprising that the negative effects associated with urbanization are increasing concerns that attract the attention of people around the world. Urbanization has a negative impact on the environment mainly due to modification of the chemical and physical properties of the atmosphere, pollution production, and ground cover. All the accumulated negative impacts are known as urban heat island (UHI). The UHI is understood to be a rise in the temperature of man-made regions, producing a clear "warm island" among the "cool seas" represented by lower temperatures than the nearby natural landscape. Hot islands on the spatial scale can actually be formed in urban and rural areas. Hot islands in cities are preferred because their surfaces tend to release large amounts of heat. Nevertheless, the negative impact of UHI not only affects the population in the urban environment but also humans and their ecosystems that are far from the city. UHI is indirectly related to climate change because of its contribution to the greenhouse effect. This situation will ultimately lead to global warming, the impact of which is beginning to be felt today by almost the majority of the population living in developed and developing countries [16]. The interaction between climate change and heat island effect occurs in two ways, namely, (1) the warming climate will increase higher temperatures in hot island areas, and (2) cooling strategies to reduce hot islands can help communities adapt to the effects of climate change. In addition, it can also reduce greenhouse gas emissions that cause climate change. Climate change generally causes higher temperatures and longer heat waves, more often and more severely. Therefore in urban areas that have suffered due to heat, the island will bear the brunt of this tougher heat event [17]. Furthermore, the climate change that occurs will contribute to the increase in the cost of "hot islands" for urban areas [18].

To find out how much the population feels comfortable living in Ambon city, an index is used which indicates the existence of a comfortable or uncomfortable situation by taking into account the humidity and air temperature. This index is known as the temperature humidity index (THI). Based on the editors of the *Encyclopaedia Britannica*, THI is a combination of water humidity and water that is a measure of the degree of discomfort experienced by individuals in warm weather; it was originally called the discomfort index. The THI formula is as follows:

$$\text{THI} = \text{Tdb} - [0.55 - (0.55 \times \text{RH}/100)] \times (\text{Tdb} - 58) \tag{3}$$

where Tdb (°F) is the temperature of water measured by a thermometer freely exposed to the air but shielded from radiation and moisture. It is a temperature thermometer, and it is the true thermodynamic temperature, and RH (%) is the relative humidity [19]. Besides that, there is also another THI, namely, discomfort index (DI). DI is intended to determine the inconvenience of the microclimate conditions in a place quantitatively. Basic calculation of DI also uses air humidity and air temperature data [5].

3.3 NDVI distribution and discomfort index in Ambon City

NDVI value is a value from the processing of vegetation indices from infrared satellite channels and red canals that show the level of leaf chlorophyll concentration which correlates with vegetation density based on spectral values in each pixel.

NDVI always ranges from −1 to +1, but there isn't a distinct boundary for each type of land cover. If we have negative values, it's highly likely that it's water. On the other hand, if we have a NDVI value close to +1, there's a high possibility that it's dense green leaves. In case NDVI is close to zero, there are no green leaves, and it could even be an urbanized area [20]. In other words, the distribution of NDVI shows the distribution of the amount of vegetation on a land. High NDVI values generally indicate a land cover with a lot of vegetation that will provide an atmosphere of coolness in the local environment. The vegetation index in this study is used to determine the percentage of green cover that can be assumed as a GOS from the LANDSAT-8 image so that it is expected to reflect the actual conditions in the study area. Based on the results of the analysis conducted, it shows that the higher the NDVI value, the higher the percentage value of green cover. This confirms that there is a close relationship between the value of the vegetation index and the percentage of green cover in the study area. The distribution of NDVI values in Ambon City is presented in **Figure 4**.

In general, high NDVI values in Ambon City are located in the northern part and a little in the south as shown in the area which is dark yellow to brown. Other regions have low NDVI values which indicate that there is very little vegetation in the area. The NDVI distribution consists of four levels of greenness, high, medium, low, and non-vegetated as presented in **Figure 4**, and then is overlapped with three discomfort distribution maps so that the three new maps are obtained, i.e., the NDVI map distribution and discomfort in Ambon City at 09:00–12:00 pm and 16:00 pm. The NDVI index distribution map illustrates clearly that the distribution of NDVI values is dominated by low NDVI followed by only a small number of medium NDVI in the northern and southern parts of the city. The non-vegetated area is also very small in the northwest, while high NDVI is not present.

The comfort level of an area is an indicator used in UGS planning in an urban area. Change in climate elements, namely, the increasing air temperature, is the most direct factor that can be felt and affect the level of human comfort [21]. Quantitatively, the comfort level of an area can be approached with various

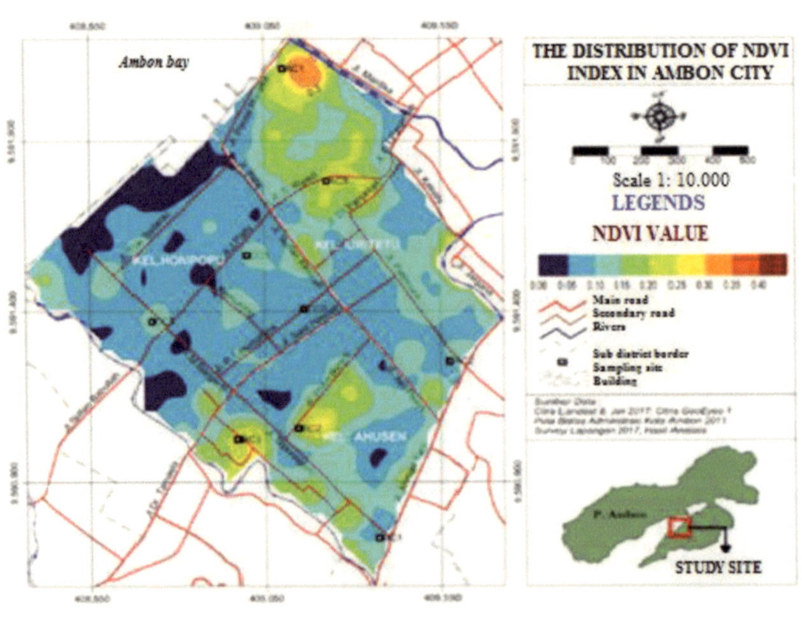

Figure 4.
The distribution of NDVI values in Ambon City.

Code of demonstration plot	Value of discomfort index at			
	09:00 pm	12:00 pm	16:00 pm	Remarks
A1	27.9	28.5	28.6	
A2	28.1	29.6	29.3	
A3	28.4	30.0	28.4	
B1	28.1	29.1	27.8	
B2	27.3	28.5	27.2	
B3	25.4	29.5	28.6	
C1	26.7	28.8	29.2	
C2	28.3	29.9	27.5	
C3	28.4	30.2	28.7	
Average	**27.6**	**29.3**	**28.4**	

Table 4.
Distribution of discomfort index value in Ambon City.

approaches. One of them is DI as implemented in this research. In addition to air temperature, comfort is influenced by other climate parameters and subjects who feel comfortable. A climate parameter that also affects human comfort is wind. The results of temperature measurements and the humidity of the green open space area of the city of Ambon in nine sampling locations showed different values based on the analysis of inconvenience index (DI) for the morning interval (at 09:00 pm); during the day (12:00 pm) and evening (16:00 pm) as presented in **Table 4**.

From **Table 4**, there are three new maps that describe the distribution of DI, which are discomfort map in Ambon City at 09:00–12:00 pm and 16:00 pm. Based on the results of interviews with 150 respondents in 9 sampling locations, 141 people fit the inconvenience as stated on the map, and 9 people stated that they did not match the distribution map of DI. Thus, this confirms that the making of the distribution map of DI is in accordance with the reality in the field regarding the discomfort felt during occupying in Ambon City. These three maps are then one-by-one overlaid with the map of the distribution of NDVI index so that the NDVI distribution index map and discomfort in Ambon City at 09:00–12:00 pm and 16:00 pm are obtained. The map is presented in **Figures 5–7**.

The majority condition of DI 70% is in the low NDVI and is followed by DI 60% in the southern part of the city (**Figure 5**). This situation shows that in the morning alone, more than 50% of the city population does not feel comfortable. In other words it may lead to physical symptoms and also influence mental health. The existence of medium NDVI is also due to too little area, so it cannot provide significant comfort for city residents.

DI conditions that rose sharply to DI 80% were in low NDVI, and those that remained were DI 70% only in the north especially near medium NDVI (**Figure 6**). This condition shows that during the day, medium NDVI plays a small role in maintaining a level of DI 70%. Although in the southern part of the city, two NDVI medium areas were found, they were found unable to maintain DI 60% in the area as shown at 09:00 pm in the morning. This condition illustrates that urban residents are increasingly uncomfortable as indicated by the increase DI 80%.

The condition in the evening at 16:00 pm remains the same as the condition at 09:00 pm in the morning (**Figure 7**). However, DI 80% still remains, especially in the western part of the city. The area of DI 60% which was originally in the south

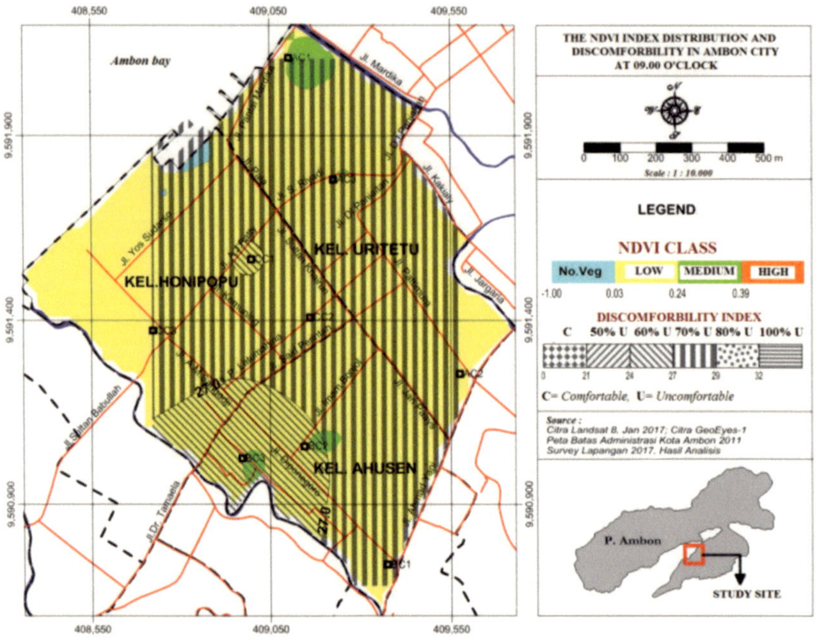

Figure 5.
The NDVI index distribution and discomfort in Ambon City at 09:00 pm.

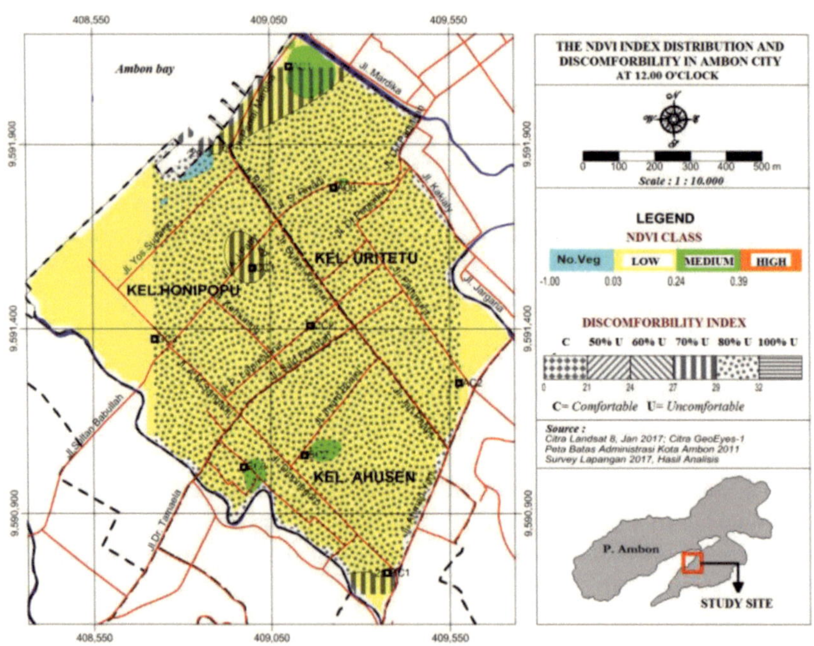

Figure 6.
The NDVI index distribution and discomfort in Ambon City at 12:00 pm.

at 09:00 pm turned out at 16:00 pm it remained at DI 80%. This shows that there is no change in discomfort at all. Through the three NDVI distribution index maps and discomfort in Ambon City (at 09:00–12:00 pm and 16:00 pm), we can find out which areas have high and low vegetation. Thus we can plan which areas need to be planted with vegetation, both grasses and trees, including how wide the building needs to be planted. Thus, in general, Ambon City residents feel uncomfortable.

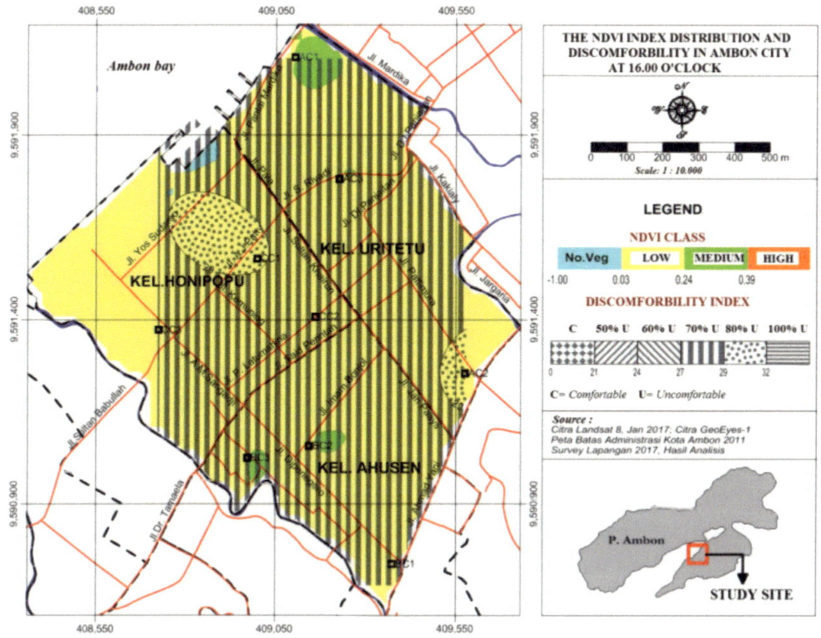

Figure 7.
The NDVI index distribution and discomfort in Ambon City at 16:00 pm.

Real effort is needed to carry out adaptations and mitigations in both the urban center and the environment. Based on the experience of daily living in European countries and Indonesia, the inconvenience is certainly felt more by developed countries than developing countries. Of course because of the people who have enjoyed abundant prosperity so that there is a small disturbance, there will be more complaints than people from developing countries.

Spatial analysis in GIS applications has supported in urban spatial planning. Good planning in the procurement of GOS in Ambon City can provide better comfort in the future. The more limited land for GOS due to development in urban areas has urged the application of the concept of green infrastructure, especially in every implementation of development. It is realized that the government of Ambon City has not had much in the development of green infrastructure such as green roofs, green facades, green walls, etc. This is certainly very different from urban planning in developed countries such as Switzerland, the United States, France, Canada, etc. that have intensively carried out the construction of green roofs, green facades, and green walls. Furthermore, green roofs are constructed for multiple reasons, for example, for architectural features or to achieve particular environmental benefits (improved diversity species, storm water capture and retention, insulation of a building against heat gain or loss, etc.). In addition to the green roof, the green facade and green wall are also known. A green facade is created by growing climbing plants up and across the facade of a building, either plants grown in garden beds at its base or by container planting installed at different levels across the building. A green wall is made up of plants grown in supported vertical systems that are generally attached to internal or external walls, although in some cases it can be freestanding. Green walls differ from green facades in that they incorporate multiple containerized plantings to vegetation cover rather than being reliant on fewer numbers of plants that climb and spread to provide cover. They are also known as vertical gardens or living walls or bio-walls [22]. Hopefully, the government of Ambon City in the future will be able to provide wider GOS and begin to apply the concept of green infrastructure in every implementation of development.

4. Conclusion

Ambon City has really been affected by climate change. Extreme rainfall that occurs in the rainy season has triggered big flooding and has been detrimental to city residents. The impact of the flood caused a huge loss of city residents. This is due to the expansion of settlements in the protected forest area of Gunung Sirimau, the construction of houses on steep slopes, as well as the impact of littering, etc. Conversely, very hot weather in the dry season makes the city residents uncomfortable. In Ambon City it was considered less comfortable as felt by residents because of the limitations of GOS. In this case, a solution needs to be sought, among others, by providing a wider area of GOS and starting to apply the concept of green infrastructure in each development implementation in Ambon City. In addition, the adequacy of GOS in Ambon City can be known by spatial analysis in GIS. With the support of NDVI distribution maps, DI maps for observations at 09:00–12:00 pm and 16:00 pm, and overlays of thematic maps, areas that are high in DI and areas that are still lacking in vegetation can be seen including how big the area is. This research is important because it can be used as preliminary study to see the development of GOS associated with DI in Ambon City. Similar research on a regular basis or time series will be able to know the development of GOS and DI in the future.

Acknowledgements

Acknowledgments are addressed to the Ministry of Research and Technology and Higher Education, Republic of Indonesia, that has helped fund research through research scheme *Produk Terapan*, year 2017.

Conflict of interest

We (Gun Mardiatmoko and Jan Willem Hatulesila) as the authors of the paper entitled "Effects of Climate Change on City Life: Case Study in the City of Ambon, Indonesia East Region" hereby declare that there is no conflict of interest in making this paper.

Author details

Gun Mardiatmoko* and Jan Wilem Hatulesila
Forestry Department, Faculty of Agriculture, Pattimura University, Ambon, Indonesia

*Address all correspondence to: gum_mardi@yahoo.com

References

[1] Utomo. Komponen Perancangan Arsitektur Lansekap. Jakarta: Bumi Aksara; 2009

[2] Peace Corps. 1990. Reforestation in the Pacific Islands. Available from: http://www.nzdl.org. [Accessed: 24 July 2018]

[3] ArcGIS. What is NDVI (Normalized Difference Vegetation Index)? 2018. Available from: https://gisgeography.com/ndvi-normalized-difference-vegetation-index/. [Accessed: 19 March 2018]

[4] Marwoto Ginting R. Penyusunan Data dan Karakteristik Daerah Tangkapan Air Danau Sentani, Kabupaten Jayapura serta perubahan Penutupan Lahannya Menggunakan Data Penginderaan Jauh. In: Dalam Berita Inderaja Vol VIII. 2009. Bidang Penyajian Data, Pusat Data Penginderaan Jauh Lembaga Penerbangan dan Antariksa Nasional. Jakarta

[5] Fandeli C, Muhammad. Prinsip Prinsip Dasar Mengkonservasi Lanskap. Yogyakarta: Gadjah Mada University Press; 2009

[6] Climate-Data. 2017. Climate Ambon. Available from: https://id.climate-data.org/asia/indonesia/maluku/ ambon-3614/ [Accessed: 19 December 2018]

[7] BBC Indonesia. Korban banjir Ambon bertambah, ribuan rumah masih terendam. 2012. Available from: www.bbc.com. [Accessed: 22 December 2018]

[8] Patty RR. Banjir rendam puluhan rumah warga di Ambon. 2012. Available from: Regional.kompas.com. [Accessed: 28 November 2017]

[9] BBC Indonesia. Delapan tewas akibat banjir di Ambon. 2013. Available from: www.bbc.com. [Accessed: 22 December 2018]

[10] Maluku Post. Pemkot Ambon data kerusakan bencana alam. 2016. Available from: www.malukupost.com. [Accessed: 22 December 2018]

[11] Siwalima. BMKG: Curah hujan akan terus meningkat. 2017. Available from: http://www.siwalimanews.com/post/bmkg_curah_hujan_akan_terus_meningkat. [Accessed: 22 December 2018]

[12] BAPPEDA Maluku. The Disaster Thematic Map of Maluku Province. Ambon, Indonesia: The Maluku Development Planning Agency; 2017

[13] Nara OD. Analisa kecenderungan curah hujan terhadap distribusi data ekstrim pada daerah aliran sungai di Pulau Ambon. JURNAL LOGIC. 2017;**17**(1):1-8. MARET 2017. Available from: http://ojs.pnb.ac.id/index.php/LOGIC/article/view/501/438. [Accessed: 28 November 2017]

[14] Laurie. Pengantar Kepada Arsitektur Pertamanan (terjemahan). 1986. Intermata. Bandung

[15] Hakim R, Utomo H. *Komponen Perancangan Arsitektur Lansekap. Prinsip, Unsur dan Aplikasi Desain*. Jakarta: Buku. Bumi Aksara; 2003. p. 287

[16] Arrau CP, Peña MA. The Urban Heat Island (UHI) Effect. 2015. Available from: http://www.urbanheatislands.com/. [Accessed: 06 July 2016]

[17] US EPA. Climate Change and Heat Islands. 2017. Available from: https://www.epa.gov/heat-islands/climate-change-and-heat-islands. [Accessed: 07 January 2018]

[18] Castell J. Climate change contributing to urban 'heat islands' raising costs for cities. 2017. Available from: http://www.cbc.ca/news/

technology/climate-change-cities-heat-islands-1.4136194. [Accessed: 09 February 2018]

[19] Bilby T. How Do I Determine?: How do I Calculate Temperature-Humidity Index (THI)? 2014. Available from: https://www.progressivedairy.com/topics/herd-health/how-do-i-determine-how-do-i-calculate-temperature-humidity-index-thi. [Accessed: 04 January 2018]

[20] GisGeography. What is NDVI (Normalized Difference Vegetation Index)? 2018. Available from: https://gisgeography.com/ndvi-normalized-difference-vegetation-index/ [Accessed: 29 December 2018]

[21] Irwan SNR. Study on Human Thermal Comfort and Human Activity in the Tree-Shaded Areas in the Green Space of the Tropical Country. Case Study: The Prambanan Park, Yogyakarta, Indonesia. Bulletin of Chiba University, Japan; 2007

[22] Growinggreenguide. Green facade definition. 2014. Available from: http://www.growinggreenguide.org/technical-guide/introduction-to-roofs-walls-and-facades/green-facade-definition/. [Accessed: 21 June 2015]

Chapter 2

Investigating Effects of Climate Change on Health Risks in Nigeria

Ilevbare Femi Monday

Abstract

Climate change has become a major challenge globally. Human activities have several direct and indirect impacts on health. In Nigeria, the impacts of climate change are more devastating due to their vulnerability and low coping capability. Studies on the impacts of climate change on health risks in Nigeria are scare. With this rationale, this study investigates the effects of climate change on health risks in Nigeria. Evidence abounds that climate change impacts in Nigeria arise from climate change-related causes such as increase in temperature, rainfall, sea level rise, extreme weather events and, especially, increased health risks. Health risks such as cerebra-spinal meningitis, cardiovascular respiratory disorder of elderly, skin cancer, malaria, high blood pressure and morbidity were identified as the direct consequences of climate change. The study concluded that government should raise awareness on adverse effects of climate change which is common among vulnerable groups, like women, children and rural dwellers in Nigeria.

Keywords: climate change, environment, health risks, Nigeria, vulnerability

1. Introduction

Over the years, human beings have relied on the environment for existence and sustenance in a way that man's survival is determined by his interaction with the environment brought about by the activities of man. One of the global events that arise from man-environment transaction is climate change. Climate change has become the subject of debates and discourse among scholars and experts, making it one of the most topical issues in the world agenda today. According to Odey (2012), scientific evidence has revealed that climate change is an all-encompassing threat and is considered the most serious ecological threat to the survival and sustainable development of humanity.

2. What is climate change?

Climate change can refer to a change in climate, attributed directly or indirectly to human activities such as burning, farming, mining and others that have the propensity to alter the atmospheric composition of the earth and to lead to global warming [1]. Climate change has been coined as an increase in average global temperature, which is caused by natural events and human activities. However, the Intergovernmental Panel on Climate Change [2], Fourth Assessment Report (AR4), gave the most accepted definition of climate change, stipulating that 'climate change is a change in the state of the climate that can be identified by using statistical tests by changes in the mean and variability of its properties, and that persists for an extended period typically decades on longer'. According to Odjugo [3], climate change is different from the generally known terms like climatic fluctuations or climatic variability. Climatic fluctuation or variability refers to variations in the mean state and other statistics such as standard deviations of the climate on all spatial and temporal scales beyond that of individual weather events. However, climate change, like variability, may be due to natural internal processes within the climate system (internal variability) or variations in natural or anthropogenic external forces (external variability).

3. Causes of climate change

The major causes of climate change are either natural or anthropogenic factors. According to Rasak [4], the natural factors are the astronomical and the extraterrestrial factors. These astronomical factors are the changes in the eccentricity of the earth's orbit, changes in the obliquity of the plane of ecliptic and changes in orbital precession while the extraterrestrial factors include solar radiation quantity. The anthropogenic factors in climate change are directly linked to man-environment transactions whose consequences result in the emission of large amount of greenhouse gases into the atmosphere that depletes the ozone layer or activities that reduce the amount of carbons absorbed from the atmosphere.

Researchers have provided evidence that for the past decades, anthropogenic factors such as urbanization, deforestation, population growth, industrialization and the release of greenhouse gases are major factors responsible for the depletion of the ozone layer [5, 6]. However, several studies have identified Africa as the most vulnerable to the impacts of climate change [7]. This reason is not far-fetched due to the fact that developing countries in Africa have experienced and are vulnerable to the impact of climate change because of access to limited climate information, institutions, financial resources and limited adaptation capacity [8]. Nigeria as one of the most populous nations with 173 million people in Africa is not exempted [9]. Nigeria has been adversely affected by climate change due to its vulnerability and low coping capacity [10]. Also, the peculiarity of the country as one of the leading exporters of crude oil faces the danger of balancing global energy demands and engulfs on the need to address climate change and environmental considerations [11].

One major event revolving around climate change in Nigeria is the drying up of Lake Chad. The southern part of Lake Chad is the part of the section of the lake that lies inside Nigerian territory. Some years back, Lake Chad covered an estimated area of over 40,000 km, while presently it now covers 1300 km^2 [10]. The implication of this occurrence is that the land is laid to wastages by rising temperature which leads to the southwards expansion of the Sahara desert. Hence, farmlands and surrounding villages have become barren due to the overpowering nature of advancing desertification, whose ripple effects have led to the massive migration of people in search of more fertile land.

Adepoju [9] posited that the impacts of climate change in Nigeria include rising temperature, more intense and frequent weather events and sea level rise. Due to Nigeria's population, the consequences are increased water and food shortages, higher exposure to heat stress and ultraviolent radiation [9]. In support of this assertion, Borokinni [12] provided evidence that climate change events affect all aspects of human life, especially the social and environmental determinants of health, clean air, safe drinking water and food security. Thus, climate change has a lot of implications on human health. Climate and weather conditions have been identified as precursors to factors that affect human health [10]. The effect of climate change on human health has been demonstrated in literature. For instance, Nwoke et al. [13] have linked climate change to higher temperatures, which enhance production of various secondary pollutants and, thereafter, increase in the frequency of allergic and cardio-respiratory disorders and deaths caused by these air pollutants. Furthermore, cases of mental health and population mobility are a result of environmental disasters such as flooding, rising sea levels and shortages of water. Horton and McMichael [14] have identified emotional stresses and mental health problems in response to perception and fear of climate change to constitute health challenge to affected communities. In lieu of this development, the goal of this chapter is to explore the effects of climate change on health risks in Nigeria.

4. Climate change and health risks in Nigeria

Evidence has established that people's health can be affected by climate change [15]. Therefore, vulnerable populations such as young children, pregnant women, older adults, individuals with chronic sickness and disabilities and individuals with fewer resources have been identified to be at increased risk [15]. Furthermore, Hathaway and Maibach [15] have found that among vulnerable people in Asia and Africa, awareness of increasing health harms due to specific changing climatic conditions is high. The consequences of climate change on human health, especially, in Nigeria could be direct and indirect. Omoruyi and Onafalujo [16] explained that one of the direct consequences of climate change in Nigeria includes cerebra-spinal meningitis, cardiovascular respiratory disorder of the elderly people, skin cancer, high blood pressure, malaria, cholera and child and maternal health issues.

5. Cerebra-spinal meningitis and climate change

Cerebra-spinal meningitis is one of the infectious diseases likely to be caused by climate change. Incidences of meningitis, for instance, have been on the rise in Nigeria due to excessive heat. According to Akingbade [17], cases of meningitis have been reported to have increased in Nigeria as a result of excessive heat. The World Health Organization has revealed that 35% of reported meningitis outbreaks in Africa between 1996 and 2010 are from Nigeria, with statistics showing 95% of this disease happening in the northern region of Nigeria [18]. Meningitis is a disease caused by an infection due to bacteria, viruses and protozoa, of the meanings which is the thin lining that surrounds the brain and the spinal cord. Cursory investigations found that over 200 people were killed by meningitis in Nigeria and neighbouring Niger Republic within a week. Statistics revealed that there were 25,000 suspected cases and 1500 deaths in the first quarter of 2009 [17].

Abdussalam et al. [18] in an empirical investigation examined the impact of future climate change on meningitis risk in northwest Nigeria by forcing an empirical model of meningitis with monthly simulations of 7 meteorological variables from an ensemble of 13 statistically downscaled global climate model projections from phase 5 of the Coupled Model Intercomparison Experiment (CMIP5) for representative concentration pathway (RCP) 2.6, 6.0 and 8.5 scenarios, with the numbers representing the globally averaged top-of-the-atmosphere radiative imbalance (in Wm22) in 2100. The results suggest future temperature increases due to climate change have the potential to significantly increase meningitis cases in both the early (2020–2035) and late (2060–2075) twenty-first century, and for the seasonal onset of meningitis to begin about a month earlier on average by late century, in October rather than November. However, Abdussalam et al. [18] suggest that this outcome represents the climatological potential for increased cases due to climate change, as it is assumed that current prevention and treatment strategies will remain similar in the future.

Brenda et al. [19] in an empirical analysis reported that between December 2016 and May 2017, a total of 14,280 suspected meningitis cases were reported across 23 of the 36 states in Nigeria. There were 1145 deaths (8% case fatality rate) among suspected cases. The northern states Zamfara and Sokoto were at the epicentre of the meningitis epidemic in Nigeria.

6. Vector-borne diseases, infection and climate change

Climatic conditions have been shown to affect water-borne diseases in Nigeria [12]. The changes in climatic conditions are germane to lengthen the transmission seasons of important vector-borne diseases and alter their geographic range. Malaria has been identified to be caused by climate conditions caused by a unicellular organism known as Plasmodium and transmitted by the bite of infected female Anopheles mosquitoes. Evidence shows that malaria accounted for over 45% of all outpatients and about 50% of the Nigerians suffer from at least one episode of malaria each year [20].

Scholars have argued that global warming, a consequence of climate change, could be linked—directly or indirectly—to the persistence as well as the re-emergence of malaria epidemics [20, 21]. The association between climate change and malaria spread is complex and remains a subject of controversy and debates [21]. Therefore, Adewuyi and Adefemi [21] posited that the spread and severity of malaria in several places and the increased incidences of the disease in some regions could indeed be associated with the effects and consequences of climate change. With this assertion, Adewuyi and Adefemi [21] suggest that the biology of the *Plasmodium spp*, the ecology of mosquitoes and even the susceptibility of humans to malaria could all be affected directly/indirectly by extreme climatic events.

The World Health Organization [11] projected that by 2070, under both high and low emissions, over 400 million people are predicted to be at risk of malaria. Also population growth can cause increases in the population at risk in localities where malaria presence is static in the nearest future. The world's most virulent infections are also highly sensitive to climate temperature, precipitation and humidity have an influence on the life-cycles of the vectors and the infectious agents [11]. The World Health Organization [22] estimates that 212 million people were infected with human malaria parasites globally with Africa accounting for about 90% of these cases in 2015. However, 18 countries together accounted for 90% of the total cases in sub-Saharan Africa with 37 million reported cases representing 29% of these cases from Nigeria alone. Research finding estimates that malaria kills over 400,000 people every year, mainly African children under 5 years of age [12]. In a study aimed to describe malaria transmission trends and analyse the impact of climatic factors on malaria transmission in the highlands of Plateau State, Central Nigeria, carried out by Nanvyat et al. [23], it was found that climatic factors are among the major determinants of malaria transmission in the highlands of Plateau state except in Jos-North LGA where the low model deviance explained (35.4%) could mean that there are important factors driving malaria transmission in the area other than climatic factors.

Similarly, Ayeni [20] has attributed the increase in population, rainfall fluctuation and urban heat cum high thermal discomfort and the problem of unhygienic environment to have contributed to the increase in malaria morbidity in Akure, Southwestern, Nigeria. Ayeni's [20] study based on an evaluation of the existing framework on malaria incidence using meteorology data between 1986 and 2008 and hospital records between 2000 and 2008 as well as relevant field studies indicate that malaria cases increased from 24,092 (of which males and females accounted for 12,477 and 11,615, respectively) in year 2000 to 62,121 (of which males and females accounted for 30,413 and 31,708, respectively) in year 2008.

In Nigeria, evidence suggests an estimated 137,600 diarrhoeal deaths in children under 15 years of age in the baseline period of 2008 [11]. Furthermore, it was reported that under a high emissions event, diarrhoeal deaths which are linked to climate change in children under 15 years of age are projected to be 9.8% of the over 76,000 diarrhoeal deaths predicted in 2030 [11].

7. Cardiovascular diseases and climate change

The World Health Organization [11] has identified air pollution as the single largest environmental health risk [24]. Thus, non-communicable diseases constitute the largest and fastest growing global health burden, with treatment costs placing a massive strain on the government and individual resources. Campbell-Lendrum and Pruss-Ustun [24] reiterated that the major causes of air pollution, and thus of a large proportion of the non-communicable disease burden, are the energy sources that currently drive our transport, electricity generation, industry and food production systems. Poor diet (high consumption of sugar, salt, saturated fat, etc.) and unhealthy lifestyle (smoking, alcohol consumption and physical inactivity) have been implicated as major risk factors of cardiovascular disease and other non-communicable diseases.

8. Skin cancer and climate change

Evidence has proven that climate change has environmental and economic consequences on human health [25]. The effects on human diseases such as skin cancer have been relatively underemphasized. There is a direct link between ultraviolet (UV) exposure from the sun and the development of malignant skin disease [25].

According to Bharath and Turner [25], ultraviolet radiation (UVR) occupies the space between visible light and X-rays on the electromagnetic spectrum. The colour violet corresponds to the shortest wavelength in visible light and UV actually means 'beyond violet' (from the Latin word ultra, meaning 'beyond'). UV light can be further subdivided in terms of wavelength: 'long wave' UV with a range of 320–400 nm is known as UV-A; 'medium wave' UV with a range of 290–320 nm is known as UV-B and 'short wave' UV with a range of 100–290 nm is known as UV-C.1. Therefore, UV-C is known to carry the most energy and is the most damaging to biological systems while UVB causes some DNA damage in the skin.

However, three most common skin cancers have been identified. These are: basal cell carcinoma (BCC), squamous cell carcinoma (SCC) and malignant melanoma (MM). Bharath and Turner [25] identified that exposure to ultraviolet radiation is recognized as a risk factor in all three types of cancer. Oripelaye et al. [26] emphasized the alarming rate of solar intensity and HIV epidemic which have progressively eroded the protective effects of melanin especially among black-skinned populations. For instance, Oripelaye et al. [26] in a retrospective study, with research settings at the Obafemi Awolowo University Teaching Hospital, Ile-Ife,

South-western, Nigeria, included as inclusion criteria the patients who were diagnosed with primary skin cancers between January 2008 and December 2017. Their study findings indicate the frequency of primary skin cancers was 1.0%. Females (58.3%) outnumbered the males (41.7%), the ratio being 1.4:1. Furthermore, the spectrum of primary skin cancers documented by this study comprised of squamous cell carcinoma (33.3%), malignant melanoma (25%), Kaposi sarcoma (15.3%), basal cell carcinoma (9.7%) and cutaneous lymphoma (6.9%). The researchers opined that melanin remains a major protective factor for skin cancers among negroids. Hence, albinism and high burden of HIV were identified risk groups for skin cancers [26]. The eradication of HIV and enhanced sun protection were suggested in order to reduce the prevalence of skin cancers among the black race.

9. Elderly health and climate change

One profound effect of climate change is among the aged persons in Nigeria. According to Aina and Adewoyin [27], the vulnerable age are particularly more at risk of climate-related diseases because of the effect of their age on their physiological and immunological compositions. Research has provided credence that the aged are more at risk of climate-related diseases because they have a lower physiological reserve, possess a slower rate of metabolism and a weakened immune system and have a higher morbidity rate [28].

To determine the effects of climate change on the trend and prevalence of climate-related diseases among the aged in an urban setting using Ikeja, Lagos, Nigeria, as a case study, two sets of secondary data—hospital records of 600 adults aged 50 and above with clinically diagnosed cases of-climate related diseases and data on climatic parameters of temperature and rainfall—were employed. The data sets were collected for the period 2001–2015. Aina et al. [27] in the study found that temperature declined over the period of study while rainfall increased. The study also showed that incidence of high blood pressure was more prevalent (43%) than any other climate-related diseases among the sampled population. This was followed by fever and respiratory diseases. Incidences of cholera and diarrhoea as well as blindness and skin diseases were relatively few. Furthermore, the study revealed that the cases of high blood pressure, fever and respiratory diseases were positively correlated with year as they showed a progressive annual increase in relation to the fluctuations in rainfall and temperature, particularly increased rainfall. Finally, the fluctuations in rainfall and temperature accounted for 11.5% of the variations in climate-related diseases among the aged in the period studied [27].

10. Mitigation measures

The mitigation and adaptive measures against the effects of climate change are very critical for Nigeria to reduce the health risks brought about by this global threat. The health sector from primary, secondary and tertiary health institutions should identify the major regional health hazards caused by climate change and ensure that the development of risk-lessening adaptations are employed. According to Borokinni [12], adaptation capacities and strategies differ among populations. Borokinni [12] elaborated that this will be particularly necessary where the rates of pre-existing disease such as childhood diarrhoea and malnutrition are already high and which would become higher due to the multiplier effects of climate change. Hence, effective adaptive strategies should involve collaboration among diverse government sectors, research institutes, various disciplines and communities.

There is the need to protect the environment; hence, there should be awareness of the potential health risks associated with climate change. Relevant agencies should create awareness among citizens including disaster and emerging workers about climate change impacts and how they affect vulnerable populations. This could be achieved by providing basic training, workshops and sensitization programmes to raise awareness and promote climate change adaptation. In addition, the longer-term global health benefits should strengthen support for such actions. The health benefits will result from mitigating actions that address modes of transportation, housing-design, energy generation and agricultural systems. Borokinni [12] emphasized that in many poor populations such as Nigeria, improvements in environment-related technologies will aid to replace indoor-polluting cooking fuels with low-carbon fuels and improvements in family planning literacy, which will lead to fewer, better spaced pregnancies. This will reduce pressures on the climate system. The effectiveness of these actions will directly reduce well-known risk factors for diseases and premature death emanating from air pollution, sedentary lifestyles and dietary excesses. Sedentary lifestyle has been linked to limited physical activity, prolonged sitting at workplace, vehicles, communities, schools and public places [29]. Sedentary behaviours are defined as those behaviours associated with lesser energy expenditure [29]. According to Mfrekemfon and Okey-Orji [29], attention has shifted from a physically demanding life to that of lesser physical activities, which has enabled individuals to be vulnerable to the high risk of having serious health ailments such as obesity, hypertension, cardiac abnormality and cancers. However, these ailments could be avoided if people shun unhealthy lifestyles. Therefore, there is the need for individuals to make conscious efforts and initiatives to engage in more physical activities, and modifying their dietary habits and avoiding unhealthy behaviour.

Innovative urban design has also been identified to have some positive advantages with regard to energy use, greenhouse gas emissions, effects of urban heat, patterns of physical activity and community cohesion. However, four strategies were identified to have the largest aggregate potential for health and SLCP mitigation benefits as well as reducing CO_2.

These strategies are: policies and investments that prioritize dedicated rapid transit and walking and cycling networks in compact cities can promote health in multiple ways, including reduced air pollution exposures, reduced injury risks and greater opportunities for safe active travel; second, promoting healthier diets rich in plant-based foods and low in red and processed meats among affluent populations at risk of a range of diet-related non-communicable diseases will have a positive effect on health; third, encouraging the use of clean and efficient cook stoves and fuels, and cleaner energy sources, in low-income households that currently rely on solid fuels for heating and cooking; fourth, reducing vehicle emissions of both particulate matter as well as ozone precursors (e.g., NO_2) by implementing stricter vehicle and fuel emissions and efficiency standards.

Furthermore, to mitigate the threats of climate change in Nigeria, reducing polluting vehicles and public transportation reduce greenhouse gases, and walking and cycling will facilitate physical activity that improves well-being among the vulnerable population. Agencies and establishments under the Ministry of Health in Nigeria should be engaged in leadership and coordination of health-related matters, especially the ones that are environmental burden diseases. Hence, they should play a dominant role in raising awareness of the health impacts of air pollution and in advocacy activities.

Nigeria is recognized as a fossil fuel-dependent economy with a large climate-sensitive agricultural sector; therefore, the development of a climate change policy and response strategy is critical. Government should invest more in low-carbon fuels and renewable energy in Nigeria. However, there should be joint efforts between the government and the citizenry in every community to combat climate change in Nigeria. In addition, relevant agencies should conduct periodic assessments of the vulnerability of populations and population groups to climate change and identify appropriate adaptation strategies. Indicators for climate and environmental health in national surveillance systems should be promoted, providing evidence to support decision-making and behaviour to reduce climate-related health risks in Nigeria. Human actions that influence climate change include pressures due to population growth and region-specific types and patterns of consumption. Therefore, it becomes imperative for households and individuals to learn how to adapt to the threats of climate change, and be ready to share information with other stakeholders about their daily experiences with climate change impacts and adaptation. In addition, individuals must be prepared to imbibe attitudinal change in order to build capacity for adaptation towards climate change.

Environmental psychologists can assist in conceptualizing and understanding better the psycho-social aspects of these driving forces behind climate change. This could be achieved by providing behavioural analyses of consumption by targeting on those behaviours that contribute the most to climate change. Hence, individual predictors of consumption that include ability (e.g., income, skills) and motivation (e.g., connection to nature, perceptions of needs versus a luxuries, core psychological needs) to engage in consumption are some of the psychological variables. Climate change can have psychosocial impacts on individuals, groups and communities due to relative risk appraisals, mental models and media representation. However, there are some psychological barriers why people do not respond adequately to the risks of climate change. Among these are ignorance, uncertainty, mistrust, denial, judgmental discounting, habits and perceived behavioural control.

11. Conclusion

The health risks associated with climate change in Nigeria cannot be overemphasized. All populations are affected by climate change, particularly the vulnerable like the children and the elderly people. The impacts of climate change are also expected to increase over the years, which mean that some existing health challenges will increase. Therefore, it is very important for everyone to have a better knowledge and perception about climate change as it affects human health. This is expected to inform people's decision-making about how to reduce the impact of the amount of climate change in the nearest future. In line with this development, environmental education and awareness should be promoted by stakeholders and government to bring about the best adaptation and mitigation mechanisms among vulnerable communities. Also, there should be workshops, seminars and forums on climate change adaptation and mitigation organized regularly in schools, universities, communities, religious houses, motor parks and public places. Research needs on climate change should be identified by the government and researchers. There is also the need for children in Nigeria to be taught the foundation of a climate-smart lifestyle, environmentally friendly behaviour and protection. Furthermore, students from primary to tertiary institutions are empowered with relevant information on how to choose professions that will assist the society to solve emerging environmental problems as a consequence of climate change in Nigeria. Adequate funding of groundbreaking researches from various multidisciplinary disciplines relating to climate change should be given priority in Nigeria. Lastly, all stakeholders should improve regional, national and local capacity to respond to public health needs during climate-related emergencies.

DOI: http://dx.doi.org/10.5772/intechopen.86912

Author details

Ilevbare Femi Monday
Department of Psychology, Faculty of Social Sciences, Obafemi Awolowo University, Ile-Ife, Nigeria

*Address all correspondence to: femilevbare@oauife.edu.ng

References

[1] Omotosho JA. Melting Ice and Climate Change: Why Should I Care? A paper delivered on the occasion marking 2007 World Environment Day Celebration; 5th June, 2007; The Ondo State Library Complex; 2007

[2] Intergovernmental Panel on Climate Change (IPCC). Climate Change 2007: The Physical Science Basis, Summary for Policymakers. Contribution of Working Group I to the Fourth Assessment Report of the Intergovernmental Panel on Climate Change. Geneva, Switzerland: Intergovernmental Panel on Climate Change; 2007

[3] Odjugo PAO. Analysis of climate change awareness in Nigeria. Academic Journals. 2013;**8**(26):1203-1211. DOI: 10.5897/SRE11.2018

[4] Rasak B. Conceptualizing the Relationship Between Climate Changes and Human Health in Nigeria: Panoply of Readings in Social Sciences; Lesson for and from Nigeria. Canaan Land, Ota: Department of Sociology, College of Development Studies, Covenant University; 2013. pp. 249-266

[5] Buba AD. Climate change and water problems in Chad Republic. Journal of Arid Environments. 2004;**3**(2):42-50

[6] Odjugo PAO. The impact of climate change on water resources, global and regional analysis. The Indonesian Journal of Geography. 2007;**39**(1):23-41

[7] Ilevbare FM, Idemudia ES. Influence of gender and age on attitudes toward climate change: A survey of a Nigerian University Students' Population. Gender and Behaviour. 2017;**15**(4):9831-9845. Available from: http://www.ajol.info/index. php/gab/article/view/165789

[8] Ojomo E, Elliot M, Amjad U, Bartram J. Climate change preparedness: A knowledge and attitudes study in Southern Nigeria. Environments. 2015;**2**:435-448. DOI: 10.3390/environments2040435

[9] Adepoju AA. Climate Change and Health in Nigeria. Nigerian Tribune. 2017. Available from: https://www.tribuneonline.com [Accessed: 20 April 2019]

[10] During R. Nigeria: Impact of Climate Change on Health in Nigeria. ThisDay Newspaper; 2017

[11] World Health Organization (WHO). Climate Change and Health: Country Profile, Nigeria. United Nations Framework Convention on Climate Change. 2015. Available from: https://www.who.who.int/globalchange/resources/PHE-country-profile-Nigeria.pdf?ua=1 [Accessed: 13 April 2019]

[12] Borokinni J. Climate Change and Health Impacts. The Nation Newspaper. 2017. Available from: https://nationonline.ng.net/climate-change-health-impacts/

[13] Nwoke BEB, Nwoke EA, Ukpai OM. Effect of climate change on human health and some adaptive strategies—A review. Bayero Journal of Pure and Applied Sciences. 2009;**2**(1):168-172

[14] Horton G, McMichael T. Climate Change, Health Check 2020. A Report by Climate Institute of Australia. 2008. Available from: www.climateinstitute.org.au

[15] Hathaway J, Maibach EW. Health implications of climate change: A review of the literature about the perception of the public and health professionals. Current Environmental Health Reports. 2018;**5**:197-204

[16] Omoruyi EP, Onafalujo AK. Effects of climate change on health risks in Nigeria. Asian Journal of Business

and Management Sciences. 2011; **1**(1):204-215

[17] Akingbade T. Climate Change effects in Nigeria: Heat, Dusty Weather Rise Health Concerns: The Guardian; 2010

[18] Abdussalam AF, Monaqhani AJ, Steinhoff DF, Dukic VM, Hayden MH, Leckebusch GC. The impact of climate change in Meningitis in Northwest, Nigeria: An assessment using CMIP5 climate model simulations. American Meteorological Society. 2014:371-379. DOI: 10.1175/WCAS-D-13-000681

[19] Brenda AK, Kwambana A, Rahab CA, Martin A. Meningococccus Serogroup C Clousal complex ST-10217 Outbreak in Zamfara State, Northern, Nigeria. Scientific Reports 8. 2018:14194. Available from: https//www.nature.com/articles/541598-018-32475-2

[20] Ayeni AO. Malaria morbidity in Akure, Southwest, Nigeria: A temporal observation in a climate change scenario. Trends in Applied Sciences Research. 2011;**6**:488-494

[21] Adewuyi EO, Adefemi K. Climate change and malaria control: the importance of mitigation and a call to actions. International Journal of Community Medicine and Public health. 2016;**3**(4):770-775. DOI: 10.18203/2394-6040.ijemph20160911

[22] World Health Organisation. World Malaria Report. Geneva: World Health Organisation; 2016

[23] Nanvyat N, Mulambalah CS, Ajiji BY, Dakul DA, Tsingalia HM. Malaria transmission trends and its lagged association with climatic factors in the highlands of Plateau State, Nigeria. Tropical Parasitology. 2018;**8**(1):18-23. DOI: 10.4103/TP-35-17

[24] Campbell-Lendrum D, Pruss-Ustun A. Climate change, air pollution and non-communicable diseases. Bulletin of the World Health Organization. 2019;**97**:160-161. DOI: 10.2471/BLT.18.224295

[25] Bharath AK, Turner RJ. Impact of climate change on skin cancer. Journal of the Royal Society of Medicine. 2009;**102**:215-218

[26] Oripelaye MM, Oladele AO, Olanrewaju FO, Olaofe OO. The evolving pattern of primary skin cancers in Ile-Ife, Nigeria. Serbian Journal of Dermatology and Venereology. 2018;**10**(3):90-95

[27] Aina TA, Adewoyin Y. Climate change and health of the aged in Lagos, Nigeria. Australian Journal of Basic and Applied Sciences. 2017;**11**(13):8-16

[28] Carnes BA. Impact of climate change on elder health. Journal of Gerontology. 2014;**69**:9

[29] Mfrekemfon PI, Okey-Orji S. Sedentary lifestyle: health implications. IOSR Journal of Nursing and Health Science. 2015;**4**(2):20-25

Chapter 3

Heavy Metals and the Environment

Iveta Cimboláková, Ivan Uher, Katarína Veszelits Laktičová, Mária Vargová, Tatiana Kimáková and Ingrid Papajová

Abstract

Global environmental contamination is one of the most significant environmental problems in contemporary society. Pollutants are entering the environment from different sources, and on the basis of their physico-chemical properties, they are transported and participate in biochemical cycles in the varied components of the environment, namely in the air, aquatic environment, soil and in rocks or segments. They enter the food chain through which they enter the human body, where they are transformed into either harmless metabolites (detoxification) that are easily excluded or else harmful, reactive products are formed. Heavy metals are one of the most dangerous groups of biologically important pollutants. The burden of the environment puts more significant burden on populations and ecosystems. They form integrant part of the earth's surface and therefore are present throughout the land. We can utter that contamination of the environment and its consequences for living organisms have long been in forefront of the interest in scientific as well as lay community.

Keywords: environment, heavy metals – Cd, Hg, risks of environmental pollution, food chain, health

1. Introduction

Modern civilization process brings on the one hand, better living standards, on the other hand, it has negative side effects in the form of impaired ecological, biological and natural conditions of life. Global environmental contamination is one of the most significant environmental problems at present. It is associated with an unprecedented boom in the utilization of chemicals in industrial and agricultural production. As a result, there is a relatively high concentration of toxic substances in the environment. These substances are not natural and are "strange" and „unfriendly "to the environment. Contaminants can be organic or anorganic compounds that are not naturally found in the environment; e.g., xenobiotics which can be found in unnaturally high concentrations (e.g. heavy metals) in individual environmental segments. The attention of professionals and lay public is mainly focused on hazardous substances, i.e. those that are difficult to decompose in natural surroundings, with high persistence and often exhibiting toxic effects on the environment [1–3].

Effects of environmental stress - sensitivity of a given organism to a certain stressor depends on its state of development and the conditions of its metabolism.

IntechOpen

When humans are concerned, especially the fetus, the newborn and the mother during pregnancy should be protected. Sick, weakened or weak individuals react very sensitively to environmental pollution. Smog disasters threaten humans and animals, and soil changes adversely affect vegetation. Very often not one, but several factors stress and pollute the environment. The simultaneous action of multiple factors may be substantially different than in the case of an individual effect; antagonistic, summative, synergistic, potentiating effects are recognized in these cases. It is true that the responses of biological system to environmental pollution can be: *individual-level responses* - (metabolic disorders stimulation or inhibition depending on stress level), production of chemical stress agents, changes in hormone levels (vertebrate adaptation syndrome), reproductive disorders, impaired orientation and even death in cases of extreme stress, *population-level responses* - extinction of sensitive individuals, change in size and age structure of the population, strong selection of genetically resistant individuals, general decline in genetic diversity within the population, extinction of populations, *biocenosis and ecosystem level responses* - change in competition and predator - prey-victim ratio, change in the field of parasitism and disease, change of species spectrum and elimination of sensitive species and spreading of resistant species, decline in biomass and diversity of species, change of closed metabolism system into an open one (partial or complete loss of minerals from natural deposits), change from equilibrium to imbalance, from ecosystem stability to instability, collapse of biocoenosis (in extreme cases). Toxic substances are particularly environmentally harmful to animal and human health, and thus, health risk assessment methods are particularly important in this respect.

Climate change, water, soil and health. *Climatic conditions* in Europe but also on other continents are changing. As a result of these changes, extreme weather-related events (floods, heat waves, droughts, forest fires, changes in vegetation, changes in the sea and ocean levels) are becoming more and more frequent. The change of the global climate, its impacts, and the need for solutions represent one of the most important and widely discussed environmental issues in human history so far. This change can be triggered by a number of internal and external factors, including human activity. Key effects caused by anthropogenic activity are the changes in greenhouse gas concentrations, ozonosphere disruption, local air pollution, land use and countryside exploitation. Given the complexity of the whole system, at present, it is extremely difficult to quantify precisely the human share on the total climate change. Subsequent assessment of the health consequences of the climate change is still relatively problematic, as most human health disorders are caused by several factors and take place against the backdrop of economic, social, demographic and overall environmental changes. *The area of climate change, water and soil - international commitments* - The UN Framework Convention on Climate Change, adopted in 1992 in New York, has become the basis for tackling climate change at international level. Its ultimate goal is to stabilize the impacts of the concentration of greenhouse gases in the atmosphere at a level that would prevent the dangerous consequences of human interaction and the Earth's climatic system. In 1997, the Kyoto Protocol to the Convention was adopted to tighten up the commitments of individual countries (officially adopted in 2005). This is the first binding UN legislation in the area of environment. Already in 1979, at the UNECE Convention in Geneva, the so-called "Convention on Long Range Transboundary Air Pollution„ was signed. The basic aim is to protect the environment from air pollution respectively its gradual reduction. The Convention was supplemented by additional protocols related to the long-term funding of the Cooperative Programme for Monitoring and Evaluation of the Long-range Transmission (Geneva, 1984, Oslo, 1994), reduction of sulfur emissions or their transboundary flows (Helsinki, 1985), reduction of nitrogen oxide emissions or their flows crossing the borders (Sofia, 1988), limiting the emissions of volatile organic compounds - VOCs (1991), reducing emissions of persistent organic pollutants, reducing acidification, eutrophication and ground-level ozone. In the context of water protection at international level, already in 1972, the European Council proclaimed the European Water Charter, which highlights the vital importance of water and the inevitable need to protect and use water resources. "the Directive no. 2000/60/EC of the European Parliament and Council", establishing the framework for the Community action in the field of water policy (WFD), which entered into force in 2000, provides the legislative framework for the introduction of a single policy in the countries of the European Union. Nowadays, the issue of water cleanliness and protection seems to be a priority, not only from a general and economic point of view, but above all from the fact that the quantity and quality of water is an essential factor in protecting and creating the environment [3–7].

2. Atmosphere

The word *atmosphere* comes from Greek (atmos -vapor, sfaira - sphere) and represents the gaseous layer around the Earth. It protects us from harmful cosmic radiation, harmful sunlight, solar winds and is the place where weather is created. There could be no life without the atmosphere. Gases forming the atmosphere are retained around the Earth by gravitational force. *The composition and properties of air*: Air is an essential component of the biosphere, without which the existence of various forms of life on Earth would not have been possible. The gases that create the atmosphere are kept around the Earth by gravitational force. The basic elements of the atmosphere are nitrogen (78.1%), oxygen (20.9%), argon (0.9%) and carbon dioxide (0.033%). The secondary components are noble gases (He, Kr, Ne, Xe), hydrogen, ozone, nitrogen oxides, ammonia, methane, iodine. The atmosphere provides protection from harmful cosmic radiation, harmful sunlight and solar wind. It has no significant upper boundaries, as it merges with space and rotates with the Earth. It is an essential condition for life as it transforms the radiant energy of the Sun, regulates the distribution of humidity and heat, and affects the spatial arrangement of the entire landscape. Based on the temperature-to-height dependence, the Earth's air cover is divided into individual layers: the troposphere, the stratosphere, the mesosphere, the thermosphere, and the exosphere. *The troposphere* (from the Greek tropos - change) is the lowermost and the densest part of the atmosphere and makes up to 80% of its weight. It reaches 16–18 km above the equator, 8–10 km above the poles and 11 km in the temperate zone. With height, its temperature drops by an average of 0.65°C to 100 m. The temperature of this atmosphere layer is about 17 to −52°C. The composition of troposphere is quite constant. It contains about 78% nitrogen, 20% oxygen, small amounts of other gases and also contains virtually all water vapor. The troposphere is the most important layer of the atmosphere for life, with clouds being formed there and the occurrence of the majority of weather-related phenomena. *The Stratosphere* (from the Latin stratum - blanket) is the second major layer of the Earth's atmosphere after the troposphere. It reaches a height of 45–50 km above the Earth. About 20–30 km above the Earth's surface, the stratosphere contains ozone, which is called stratospheric ozone. It acts as a filter, trapping harmful ultraviolet radiation, and transmitting life-giving light and heat to the Earth. It completely absorbs UV-C radiation, which has lethal effects on the living organism and partially absorbs the short-wave UV-B radiation (wavelength of 280–315 nm), which is capable of causing many adverse effects. Although ozone in the stratosphere is naturally created and destroyed in a constant, balanced rate, people are gradually breaking this balance by using ozone-consuming substances. Increased penetration of UV-B radiation through the ozone layer increases the risk of skin cancer, cataracts and also contributes to immune system disruption. In addition, it damages crops such as soybeans, beans, disrupting the food chain in the oceans as well. *Ozone* also occurs in the lower part of the atmosphere as tropospheric ozone. Ozone in the ground level atmosphere has a harmful effect on living organisms. Unlike stratospheric ozone, tropospheric ozone does not protect organisms but, on the contrary, damages the respiratory organs of plants and animals. In recent decades, "good" stratospheric ozone has been decreasing and "bad" tropospheric ozone has been increasing. Air conditioners, fire extinguishers and chemicals such as Freon used in refrigerators and freezers can get to the stratosphere where they decompose and the released bromine and chlorine molecules thus destroying "good" ozone. One molecule of chlorine or bromine can destroy up to 100,000 ozone molecules, so ozone in the stratosphere disappears faster than it can naturally be supplied. Volcano explosions contribute only with a tiny amount, about 3% of the total, of chlorine to the stratosphere, while people contribute with 82%. *The mesosphere* extends to a height of about 80 km. This atmosphere layer is characterized by a temperature drop down to −90°C, which represents the lowest temperature area in the whole atmosphere. The reason for the temperature drop is extremely thin air and the near absence of ozone. It should also be noted that in the mesosphere the temperature varies depending on the season of the year. The boundary within the mesosphere is known as mesopause. Most of the meteorites falling onto Earth mostly burn in the mesosphere. *The ionosphere* represents the ionized part of the atmosphere that affects the propagation of electromagnetic signals. Located between 80 and 600 km in the mesosphere and thermosphere, it consists of neutral gas, ions and electrons. *The thermosphere* extends to the height of 690 km. The temperature rises with increasing height. It reaches up to 1500°C at a height of around 300 km and is no longer changing at higher altitudes. The thermosphere has the lowest density, it contains only 0.001% of the mass of the whole atmosphere. *The exosphere* is sometimes not even distinguished as a separate layer but is assigned to the thermosphere. It represents the highest layer of the atmosphere, more than 800 km above the Earth's surface. In the exosphere, conditions for the release of atmospheric particles into the interplanetary space arise [8–10]. *Air Contamination, Causes, Consequences:* The air that mankind has not been paying attention to (and did not have to pay) in the past, is nowadays becoming an acute and widely discussed issue. Since air is not inexhaustible. Its pollution is more perceptible from year to year. There are always new ways and means of its pollution, which also affect their originators, people, animals and nature. *A pollutant* is any substance introduced by human activity directly or indirectly into the air that has or may have harmful effects on human health or the environment, except for a substance the introduction of which into the environment is governed by a specific regulation. *Emission* is any direct or indirect release of a pollutant into the air. A *stationary source of air pollution* is a technological complex, warehouse or landfill of fuels, raw materials and products, waste dump, quarry or other area with the possibility of steaming, burning or polluting or other construction, object, equipment and activity that pollutes or can pollute the air; it is defined as the sum of all facilities and activities within a functional unit and a spatial unit. A *mobile source of air pollution* is a mobile device with an internal combustion engine or other propulsion engine that pollutes the air. The air is polluted by the discharge of various substances into the atmosphere and the processes taking place directly in the air. The atmosphere is under increasing pressure from greenhouse gases, which represent climate change and under pressure from ozone depleting chemicals. Pollutants, including substances that cause acid rain, are often transferred over long distances, thus damaging soil and water. Air pollution is the introduction of pollutants into the atmosphere which, either directly, after a chemical change or by interaction with another substance, adversely affects the environment. We know various sources of air pollution, namely anthropogenic and natural, which include: combustion of fossil fuels in electricity generation, transport, industry and households, industrial processes and the use of solvents, for example in the chemical and mineral processing industries, agriculture, waste treatment, volcanic eruptions, windblown dust, sea salt spray, and emissions of volatile organic compounds from plants are examples of natural emission sources. Within broader understanding of air pollution, we also include harmful electromagnetic radiation, noise, heat, etc., among pollutants. The following inorganic substances pollute the air: sulfur oxidation products (sulfur dioxide, sulfur trioxide, sulfuric acid, sulfates), which are introduced into the air by the combustion and processing of coal and oil. Nitrogen oxidation products (nitrogen oxide, nitrous acid, nitrates) that enter the atmosphere as products of biological processes (bacterial activity), from combustion processes in industry and transport. Carbon monoxide is produced in combustion processes where there is insufficient oxygen supply to the burning fuel (exhaust gases of motor vehicles and air planes, heating). *Anthropogenic emissions* - beryllium (Be), cobalt (Co), antimony (Sb), selenium (Se) - arise mainly from coal combustion, nickel (Ni) and vanadium (V) are predominant in the combustion of diesel, arsenic (As), cadmium (Cd), copper (Cu) and zinc (Zn) are emitted mainly when melting non-metallic ores. Chromium (Cr) and zinc (Zn) are released from the iron and steel works. Inhalable and respirable particles, which can penetrate up to the alveoli [11], are considered to be dangerous to health. Other important substances - volatile organic compounds (VOC), polycyclic aromatic hydrocarbons (PAHs), polychlorinated biphenyls (PCBs), dioxins are measured selectively in targeted studies. In case of any harm to human health, animals and beasts by the action of pollutants, the emphasis is mainly on the effects of generally toxic, allergenic, carcinogenic, mutagenic, teratogenic substances. *Immissions* are substances that affect the soil, water, plants, animals and humanity. The composition of the air and its properties are variable, so its effect on the organism changes. In terms of place of origin, air pollution is divided into *primary and secondary*. *Primary air pollution* is the release of pollutants from the source of pollution. *Secondary air pollution* refers to chemical changes in some substances occurring in the process of spreading airborne exhalates. The level of air pollution is expressed by the instantaneous or average concentration of pollutants at a particular location and depends both on the emissions of pollutants and on the processes to which these emissions are subject in the air. This level is characterized by detected pollutant emissions. Polluted air damages the environment or its components, endangers or damages the human and animal organisms and impairs the environment by deteriorating odor, reducing visibility, etc. [2, 3, 10–13].

The Causes of Air Pollution: Increasing population and living standards, including energy requirements, are the main cause of the increase in air pollution. The global economy, which meets the demands of an advanced society, is characterized by increasing oxygen consumption and the release of gaseous, liquid and solid emissions. Depending on the volume of the polluted air, pollution can be divided into local (covering areas with units of tens of km^2 – i.e., air pollution of cities and industrial areas, changes caused by changes in local emission and meteorological conditions), regional (bottom troposphere pollution of entire territorial unit, in assessing regional air pollution, it is necessary to analyze the long-term impact and its consequences on soil, water and sensitive ecosystems) and global (pollution of the free atmosphere, changes in the composition of the atmosphere as a whole; the most serious pollutants being carbon dioxide and small particles of solid and liquid substances) [3, 9]. *Carbon dioxide* (CO_2) - the natural source of carbon dioxide emissions is the breathing of aerobic organisms, while the process leading to its natural decrease is the photosynthesis of green plants and the oceans represent the ways to absorption. The mean residence time in the atmosphere is estimated to be 2–4 years. The total CO_2 content is increasing - over the last 100 years the CO_2 concentration has increased by about 10%. The increase in CO_2 in the atmosphere is responsible for the worsening of the greenhouse effect. *Anthropogenic sources* are mainly combustion processes. Other natural processes emitting carbon dioxide include fires and volcanic activity. Carbon dioxide is emitted wherever combustion processes of carbon fossil fuels (natural gas, petroleum products, coal, coke) occur. The source of emissions is also the combustion of fuels of biological origin (biomass, wood, biodiesel and biogas). Carbon dioxide in the atmosphere absorbs the infrared radiation of the Earth's surface and thus contributes to the greenhouse effect and consequently to global warming. In higher concentrations, in poorly ventilated areas, it may exhibit toxic effects. Short-term exposure may cause headache, dizziness, difficulty in breathing, confusion immediately or with a short delay. Higher exposure may cause cramps, coma, or death. Some more serious cases of poisoning can leave brain effects, cause personality changes, and impair vision. *Carbon monoxide* - has an uncontrolled radiation impact on the atmosphere in connection with increasing methane concentration and increasing of the ozone hole. CO belongs to the photochemically active gases contributing indirectly to the greenhouse effect of the atmosphere. It is known as a precursor of ozone because it affects the formation and breakdown of ozone in the troposphere. The atmospheric residence time estimates vary, with a range of 0.1–0.3 years, some 1 month to 5 years; this also depend on the carbon monoxide removal rate. The major part of CO is formed in the atmosphere during methane oxidation, chlorophyll decomposition and terpene photooxidation. Volcanic activity, forest fires and bacterial activity in the oceans contribute to the total amount produced by natural resources. Anthropogenic activity is letting into the air from 350 to 600 million tons of CO per year. The most important emission sources include imperfect combustion, e.g. in automobiles, industry, incinerators and heating plants and incomplete combustion of carbon-containing organic substances. It is one of the most common poisons. When inhaled, it is absorbed into the lungs and re-bound to the blood dye, producing carboxyhemoglobin. CO has 200 some literature reports up to 240–300 times more affinity for blood pigment than oxygen [13, 14]. *Hydrocarbons* - the largest share is methane gas from natural resources. The second largest group is represented by terpenes from natural sources. From human activity, comes less than 5% of the total volume of hydrocarbons, of which 38.5% comes from combustion, 11.3% from solvent evaporation, 8.8% from the evaporation of crude oil and transport losses, 7.1% from refinery waste. In terms of air pollution, the combustion of hydrocarbons is of the utmost importance. When hydrocarbons enter the atmosphere as products of combustion processes, they react with the components of the polluted atmosphere or undergo photooxidation or photolysis. The most serious ones are those that create photooxid smog. Significant hazard to ozone depletion is represented by freons and halons. *Nitrous oxide* belongs to stable atmospheric components. The only source of nitrous oxide are natural processes. When converted into nitrogen, nitrous oxide represents 97% of all nitrogen compounds, remaining present in the atmosphere approximately for 4 years. Its larger part returns to the Earth's surface, of which about 6% diffuses into the stratosphere, where it disappears in photodissociation. Of the total amount of N_2O that undergoes a reaction, 98% is changed to N_2 in the atmosphere and 2% is converted to NO. *Nitric oxide* - most of it comes from natural sources. From anthropogenic activity, combustion processes (emissions from energy, municipal sources and transport) contribute significantly to NO emissions. The residence time in the atmosphere is estimated to be about 4 days. NO arises from combustion processes at sufficiently high temperatures. Under equilibrium conditions in the presence of oxygen, most NOs oxidize to NO_2, changing colorless nitric oxide to colored nitrogen dioxide. In the mesosphere and thermosphere, the photodissociation of nitric oxide is taking place, which presents the way of NO disappearance in the higher atmosphere. The photochemical conversion of NO to NO_2 can be of considerable importance for the air pollution in urban agglomerations. *Nitrogen dioxide* -Most of the nitrogen dioxide is produced directly in the polluted atmosphere by NO oxidation. Significantly less is released into air from anthropogenic sources. The removal of NO_2 from the atmosphere starts from its oxidation and hydration, resulting in nitric acid. Nitric acid in the polluted atmosphere can further react to form nitrates, which in the final phase are washed away by rain. In terms of air pollution, NO_2 photolysis, which can initiate photochemical smog, is of paramount importance. The formation and duration of photochemical smog depends on the chemical composition of the polluted atmosphere, the intensity and spectrum of the solar radiation. It is often created on warm sunny days at rush hours. *Ammonia* - the largest amounts of ammonia - are released into the atmosphere by the biodegradation of organic matter and by the reduction of nitrites or nitrates. Anthropogenic sources include the chemical industry, especially the production of fertilizers and urea and industrial waste. Ammonia gas reacts in an atmosphere with sulfuric acid, respectively nitric acid to form sulfates or nitrates. Self-cleaning processes occurring in the atmosphere such as sedimentation and rainwater rinsing allow the resulting salts to be removed from the air. The residence time in the atmosphere is estimated to be about 7 days. *Sulfur dioxide* is one of the typical and most common emission components. The largest amounts are produced by burning fossil fuels. Natural resources contribute to a lesser extent to total SO_2 emissions (emissions from volcanic activity). *Sulfur trioxide* is produced by burning fossil fuels. Small amounts get into the atmosphere due to the production of sulfuric acid, phosphate fertilizers or in galvanic plating. In the atmosphere, SO_3 reacts immediately with H_2O to form sulfuric acid. The sulfuric acid content increases with increased SO_2 concentration up to a certain critical value, from which the SO_2 content decreases further on. *Sulfane*-the main global source of sulfane emissions are natural processes such as volcanic activity and biological processes of substance degradation. Anthropogenic activity contributes to these sources only minimally, in the processes of oil, coal, pulp and paper processing. In the atmosphere, sulfate is gradually changing due to the oxidative effects of air oxygen with the contribution of solar radiation and due to the hydrolytic reactions with atmospheric moisture to form sulfuric acid. If other pollutants get into the air together with sulfate, the number of possible reactions is increased by combinations with primary and secondary pollution. *Consequences of air pollution:* ozone layer depletion (referred to as the ozone hole) is present in areas mainly above the Arctic and Antarctica with reduced ozone concentration due to anthropogenic pollution. In the ozonosphere there is a constant cycle of ozone formation and disappearance. In the presence of sunlight, photochemical processes occur, resulting in higher ozone concentrations. The most important thing concerning life on Earth is that most of the ultraviolet radiation is trapped in these processes and the visible light is transmitted to the Earth's surface. *Ozone* is a gas that is poisonous at higher concentrations. Therefore, in the troposphere where we live, it is undesirable, but in the stratosphere it is essential for life, as it absorbs dangerous UV radiation. Since 1970, we have been observing the depletion of the ozone layer around the entire globe. It is caused by civilization influences. At present, we know more than 200 chemical reactions of the ozone decomposition process. Depending on which parts of the atmosphere contain ozone, it can play a positive or negative role. *Tropospheric ozone* is ozone found in lower parts of the atmosphere, which is harmful to living organisms. Unlike stratospheric ozone, its concentration in the troposphere is increasing. Excessive ozone amount in the troposphere is as harmful as its lack in the stratosphere. Tropospheric ozone can be of stratospheric origin or is a result of complex photochemical reactions of hydrocarbons, carbon monoxide and nitrogen oxides. *Stratospheric ozone* - ozone found in the stratosphere prevents the penetration of harmful short-wave UV-B radiation with a wavelength of 280–315 nm. As a consequence of photochemical reactions in the stratosphere, besides the formation and decay of ozone, not only is there a significant attenuation of the incident solar ultraviolet radiation, but also the transmission (absorption) of energy, and thus an increase in temperature in the respective atmosphere layers. As a result of human activity, substances are released into the atmosphere, the amount of which exceeds the normal value of their occurrence in the atmosphere several times. This reduces the amount of ozone in the ozonosphere and disrupts the natural structure of the atmosphere, which permits much more UV-radiation at wavelengths that adversely affect living organisms. The stratospheric ozone layer is increasingly disrupted by the action of chlorofluorocarbons (CFCs or Freons). Freons have been developed in the 1930s, have a very wide use, are non-flammable, non-toxic, odorless, cheap and lighter than air. As a result of UV-radiation, the atoms of the halo elements (chlorine, bromine) are released, converting ozone to oxygen molecules that do not absorb UV. The decrease of ozone in the stratosphere allows ultraviolet rays to get to the Earth. Negative effects on living organisms include skin cancer, eye diseases, weakening of the immune system and others [3, 10, 13–15]. Ultraviolet rays do not only damage living organisms, but also contribute to the deterioration of plastics, wood, paper and cotton. The amount of both tropospheric and stratospheric ozone depends on the balance between the processes in which ozone is produced and the processes in which ozone is disposed of in the atmosphere. In the last quarter of the 20th century, it was found that stratospheric ozone was disappearing, while tropospheric ozone was increasing. Even though stratospheric ozone is naturally produced and destroyed by a constant, balanced rate, people are gradually disrupting this balance by using ozone-consuming substances. *Acid rain* is the result of strong air pollution, where dirt absorbed by air humidity gets back to the ground through precipitation. Rainwater with a pH value of 5.0–5.6 is slightly acidic because carbon dioxide is found in the air and absorbed by the air humidity. Acid rain is considered to be rainwater with a pH of 2.0–5.0. *The occurrence of acid rain* is mainly due to coal and oil-fired power plants, metallurgical plants, the chemical industry and transport. Sulfur and nitrogen oxides emitted by these sources combine with atmospheric moisture to form sulfuric and nitric acids. These rains have a negative impact on flora and fauna. They kill fish in lakes in bulk. Acid rain threatens plants, forests (healthy coniferous trees lose their needles after 6–8 years, sick ones after 2–3 years, only the newest needles remain on damaged coniferous trees, plant roots absorb toxins more easily in acidic environment) worms, insects and other animals that process plant remnants in healthy soil (thus enriching the soil with substances that are vital to plant life). However, if the soil is acidified by acid rain, the animals cannot live in it. Dead plant residues remain lying on the ground and no animal nutrients are formed. The food chain is disrupted. Some of the nutrients such as calcium, manganese, sodium, potassium is diluted from the soil due to the effects of acidic components of the rain; groundwater and surface water are (acidified water has a negative effect on aquatic animals and aquatic plants). Under these conditions, phytoplankton gradually disappears and due to its reduction, the light gets deeper into the water, so the water of the affected lakes is almost unnaturally clear and clean. Today, for example, only in Sweden out of 100,000 lakes, (about 20,000 are dead, lifeless), acid rains are damaging buildings, artistic and cultural landmarks. Not all sites respond to acid rain in the same way - it depends on the soil and water chemical composition. There are some sites with alkaline soil that can tolerate large doses of acid rain without significantly changing the overall pH of the environment. Acid aerosols also have a harmful effect on humans by entering the respiratory tract, irritating the mucosa and thus facilitating the entry of infections into the lungs. *The greenhouse effect* is the denotation of a phenomenon consisting of warming the lower layers of the atmosphere due to the fact that the atmosphere permits the passage of short-wave solar radiation to the Earth's surface during the day and absorbs Earth's long-wave radiation at night and thus becomes warmer. Larger wavelength heat radiation, which is emitted back from the planet's surface, is absorbed by the Earth effectively, its immediate release into space being prevented this way. The anthropogenic greenhouse effect is caused by the burning of fossil fuels, the excavation of forests, the global changes in the countryside, and contributes to global warming. Among the greenhouse gases currently having the greatest climate impact belongs carbon dioxide. It occurred naturally in the atmosphere. From 1850 to the present, its concentration increased by 27%. It is released in the burning of fossil fuels and its amount is growing due to massive deforestation too. Part of it is absorbed by the oceans and much of it by forested areas. Another significant greenhouse gas is *methane*. In the atmosphere it occurs naturally, as does carbon dioxide. It is produced by anaerobic bacteria in the digestive tract of ruminants and by the decomposition of organic matter. It is released from subsurface landfills and is also released into the atmosphere by escaping from gas pipelines. *Nitrous oxide* is a naturally occurring greenhouse gas. Its presence is increased by using nitrogen fertilizers and burning fossil fuels. *Freons* have anthropogenic origin. They are found in refrigerant gases and are part of the propellants. They disrupt the ozone layer. We are currently adding nearly 10 billion tons of carbon to the atmosphere annually. The biosphere is not capable of returning such an amount back to underground reservoirs as fossils, nor is the world ocean able to drain such an amount of carbon because of physical and chemical limitations. This is the main reason that the concentration of CO_2 but also of CH_4 in the atmosphere grows in parallel with the consumption of fossil carbon by various anthropogenic activities. *Nitrogen* is an indifferent part of the air in respect to health. Oxygen is the most important component of air, resulting from its role in respiratory physiology. The human organism is highly resistant to fluctuations in the amount of oxygen. Ozone is of little use for low concentration under natural conditions. However, it is harmful and even dangerous at high concentrations. *Carbon monoxide* is an unnatural admixture in the air. Its hygienic importance lies above all in the danger of poisoning. It is particularly dangerous because humans cannot smell it. *Sulfur dioxide* is produced by the combustion of sulfur and acts irritatingly and even as a strong poison. *Ammonia* occurs only in trace amounts in the atmosphere. It is harmful at a concentration of 0.5%, which it practically does not reach. Odorous substances are produced in an enclosed atmosphere by anthropogenic and animal activity. Further impurities in the air are e.g. mercury, and gasoline vapor, hydrogen cyanide [3, 6, 10, 14].

3. Hydrosphere

Hydrosphere (from Greek hydro - water) is a denotation that encompasses all water, whether on the surface of the Earth or bellow it and in any form... Water is the most widespread, under the surface of the Earth. Water occurs in different states and creates a discontinuous water layer of the Earth (hydrosphere). These include the waters of the oceans, seas, surface waters, and, in a broader sense, soil and groundwater, water bound in glaciers and snow, atmospheric water, and water in living organisms. on the Earth and for the animals it is directly the environment for their living. It is the main means of transporting nutrients, receiving and excreting them. Water on Earth occupies about 2/3 of its total surface area (drinking water represents about 1% of the total water; 97% saltwater contained in seas and oceans; 2% water bound in glaciers). The total water volume is about 1385 billion km^3. The origin and development of the hydrosphere is closely linked to the evolution of the rest of the Earth. Between the lithosphere, the atmosphere and the hydrosphere, there is a constant exchange of water causing changes in the chemical and isotopic composition of water. Continuous water circulation is caused by solar energy and gravity. Large (global) water cycle takes place between the ocean and the mainland, and a small water cycle arises over the oceans. In the various phases of the cycle, complex water conversion takes place [3, 6, 10]. *Meaning, function, properties and distribution of water:* The health of the population as a universal value and primary human rights represent the fundamental economic resource not only for the individual but also for the whole of society. In recent years, information has been gathering to warn of the catastrophic effects of unscrupulous industrial devastation of natural resources, water resources, and interventions in the ecological balance of flora and fauna. Water is an indispensable component of the human environment, as well as all plant and animal systems, and constitutes the basic condition of life on Earth. It is an important prerequisite for the existence of every living matter on Earth. *The importance of water for man and the environment* was accurately defined in the 12 points of the European Water Charter, proclaimed by the European Council on 6 May 1948 in Strasbourg: The Water Charter underlines the necessity to maintain sufficient water for future generations and the fact that water does not recognize state borders. Therefore, the growing water problems require international cooperation. According to data from the United Nations, polluted water kills more people than war. Up to 2 billion tons of polluted waste is discharged daily into the water worldwide. About 2 million people die of dehydration in developing countries every year on our planet, with about one in five people having no access to drinking water. More than 3000 children younger than 5 years die from diarrhea, dysentery, dehydration and cholera daily. According to the UN, about 783 million Earth inhabitants does not have access to drinking water and about 2.5 billion people do not know sanitation systems, while the quality of water resources is worse. The human body contains more than 60% water (65–75%), which is about 2/3 of the body weight. This ratio is even higher in children and newborns. Water plays an irreplaceable and irredeemable role in the life and function of the body as it participates in the digestion and metabolism, body temperature regulation, excretion of body waste, transport of oxygen and nutrients to tissues and cells. *The amount of drinking water received depends on several factors*: age, activity, environment in which a person lives, condition of the body, nutrition (composition of diet). Lack of water leads to serious damage to the human body after only a few days. In the case of excessive loss of water from the body, we feel drowsiness, weakness, confusion. Dry mucous membranes, constipation, headache, fatigue, somnolence, impaired movement coordination, pulse acceleration, drop in blood pressure and decreased performance are also *manifestations of water deficiency*. *In case of excessive fluid loss*, we are talking about dehydration. Loss of fluid above 6% can lead to collapse or death. *In the case of insufficient water supply*, harmful substances accumulate in the body, which puts the excretory organs under stress. The thicker the blood, the more difficult it becomes for the kidneys to deal with the waste. Water in tissues, blood, and lymph are thickened, weakening the immune system, failing to transmit nerve impulses, slowing cell renewal. Water is also important for thermoregulatory processes and protects the body from

DOI: http://dx.doi.org/10.5772/intechopen.86876

overheating. *Water functions*: *biological function* – it is the essential condition for the life of organisms from microorganisms to higher animals to humans, it provides nutrition for humanity, for some animal species water is their living environment, water participates in photosynthesis, it is part of components in the cell as well as regulator of thermal properties, *health preserving function* - the quality of life, hygiene, health, healing properties of mineralized and otherwise enriched waters depend on it; *economic function* – it is applied in the agricultural industry, *esthetic-cultural functions* - spas, water bodies fulfill the appropriate function, *political function* - watercourses form borders between states. *Water properties:* The physical, chemical and biological properties of water result from its structure and chemical composition. From a physical and chemical point of view, water is a very complicated compound characterized by a number of special chemical and physical properties resulting from the electron structure of its molecules. Water properties are divided into chemical, physical, microbiological and sensory. *The chemical properties of water* - water contains a wide range of chemicals, some of which are only minuscule and desirable (carbonates); others should only be present in limited quantities because they could change the color and haze properties (turbidity) of water (iron, chlorine) and there is also a group of substances undesirable in water that indicates water pollution with nitrogenous substances ((ammonia, nitrites, nitrates, phosphates, chlorides) of organic origin, etc.) [6, 14]. The chemical properties of water are determined by the content of substances dissolved in water. The main inorganic constituents of natural waters are calcium, magnesium and sodium, which are mostly present as cations such as bicarbonates, sulfates and chlorides. In natural waters, potassium, iron, manganese and small amounts of other metals are represented in small concentrations, by which the water is enriched in contact with the soil, with various minerals and rocks. From a chemical point of view, we divide the substances found in waters into inorganic and organic. From a physical point of view, these substances can be present as ionically dissolved (electrolytes), non-ionically dissolved (non-electrolytes) or as undissolved (non-miscible, miscible and buoyant or floating). *Physical properties of water*: ability to accumulate more heat; large water bodies such as lakes, seas and oceans are involved in the regulation of temperature on the Earth, electrical conductivity, which depends on ion concentration, their mobility and temperature, while the dissolved salts and gases increase the water conductivity, the water density increases from temperature of 0 to 3.98°C, at higher temperature it decreases continuously, surface tension - is the cause of capillary phenomena (capillarity of water in the soil and rocks, wetting ability, foam formation, etc.), viscosity, which together with density significantly affects hydraulic water behavior - for example, the speed of sand filtration of water depends on its value, sedimentation rate that decreases with temperature rise. Other physical properties of water include light absorption, water radioactivity, and state changes. *Biological properties of water:* The microbial recovery of natural waters consists of autochthonous (indigenous) species, for which water is the primary and natural habitat, where they participate in the circulation of substances in water and are thus reflecting natural water pollution without anthropogenic influence. Microorganisms that get into the aquatic environment by flushing from the soil, or through civilization wastes, whether communal, industrial, or agricultural, and survive for some time in this environment, represent an allochthonous (non-original) recovery, indicating not only external pollution by organic substances, but also the possibility of pathogenic germs. There are many microbial species *in natural waters.* Microbiological analyzes are carried out in a targeted manner, and indicator groups or individual species of microorganisms as indicators of water quality are selected purposefully according to ecological or hygienic criteria. Ecological classification of organisms expresses the behavior and application of organisms in certain physiological conditions and their ability to survive and adapt in new and more difficult conditions. Systematic division of organisms is done either from the perspective of their development or family relationships. This includes microorganisms, plants and animals. Ecological division relates to the participation of organisms in the circulation of substances in the aquatic environment and recognizes producers, consumers and destroyers. Producers are organisms able to assimilate inorganic nutrients and synthesize organic substances such as carbohydrates, proteins and fats from them. These include autotrophic bacteria, higher plants, algae, cyanobacteria. The source of energy is either light radiation, e.g. for algae, photosynthesis in plants or some oxidation–reduction reactions. In the case of photosynthesis, in addition to organic substances, producers also generate oxygen which can enrich water and air. Producers are the bases of aerobic life on the Earth and their photosynthesis is significantly utilized in self-purification of water. Consumers feed on finished organic substances that are processed by endoenzymes inside their bodies. Consumers include animals from protozoa to arthropods. Together with destructants they represent an organotrophic (heterotrophic) diet. Consumers release the waste substances of their metabolism into the water, especially carbon dioxide. Decomposers feed on finished organic substances. Since they do not have any food intake organs, they decompose high molecular weight substances outside of their body by exoenzymes into simpler molecules that can penetrate the cell wall into a destructive cell [3, 10, 13–15].

3.1 Division of water by origin, pollution, causes

Precipitation (atmospheric) water forms - occur in the air in the form of clouds, water vapor, precipitation and fog. This type of water is considered the cleanest, but it is contaminated by passing through polluted air layers. The greatest influence on the chemical composition of atmospheric waters has a layer of atmosphere that extends from the Earth's surface to a height of 1000–1500 m. *Surface water* - represents water that is permanently or temporarily on the surface of the Earth and is divided into: *flowing* (natural - streams, rivers, artificial - canals, conduits), stagnant (natural - seas, oceans, lakes, artificial - ponds, water reservoirs). Pollution of surface waters – the so-called "Eutrophication" is a set of natural and man-made processes leading to an increase in inorganic nutrients in water, especially nitrogen and phosphorus compounds, followed by increased growth of cyanobacteria, algae and higher plant forms, resulting in worsened ecological stability and reduced water quality. Phosphorus in surface waters comes from sewage and phosphate fertilizers used in agriculture. Nitrogen and phosphorus compounds mainly come from waste related to animal husbandry, industrial production and from sewage "water". An important source of surface water pollution is the excessive application of NPK fertilizers to the soil. It occurs mainly in stagnant, slow-flowing waters, but eutrophication can also occur in watercourses under favorable conditions (strong nutrient supply, increased water temperature and slowed flow of water). *Groundwater* is created by infiltration of rainwater and surface water into the Earth's crust. Groundwater is of fundamental importance in the hydrological cycle in supplying the population with drinking water. Groundwater pollution by nitrates is an issue that has been given increased attention in the area of groundwater protection against pollution The increased level of nitrates in groundwater is contributed to by anthropogenic activity, e.g. the application of industrial and artificial fertilizers to agricultural land, discharge of waste water from settlements and industrial buildings. Increased concentrations of nitrates in groundwater have a negative impact on both the environment and human health, since groundwater is preferably used as a source of drinking water. In particular, the prevention of groundwater pollution by nitrogen compounds is provided by integrated territorial protection of areas with potentially endangered groundwater bodies. Thus, *contamination of water resources* can be physical (occurrence of insoluble sludge and radioactive substances), chemical (water-soluble impurities), biological (germs present). Thus the pollution itself occurs by the already mentioned increased use of fertilizers and pesticide preparations, leakage of silage juices, leakage of liquid parts of fertilizers from farms, leakage of lubricating oils, fuels and so on. *Pollutants (substances contributing to pollution)* - substances directly toxic (heavy metals, cyanides, pesticides), water pollutants (dyes, oil and relates substances), substances affecting the amount of oxygen in the water (high levels of degradable substances, at the decomposition of which large quantities of O_2 in water are consumed), inert inorganic substances dissolved, undissolved, non-toxic [3, 10, 13, 14]. *Causes of water source pollution*-Man affects the quantity and quality of water resources directly through uncontrolled discharge of wastewater into watercourses or through sewerage networks. Waste water producers in the Slovak Republic are mainly industry and municipal sphere - sewerage systems of towns and villages. Inadequate purification results in high concentrations of pollutants and substances supporting the development of algae and plankton - phosphorus (P), nitrogen (N) - into the surface waters, resulting in an overall deterioration of water quality in streams and in stagnant waters (eutrophication). In the area of groundwater quality in the Slovak Republic, the issue of adverse oxidation–reduction conditions is at the forefront, which is often indicated by increased concentrations of iron (Fe), manganese (Mn), and NH_4. Almost all metals are naturally found in surface and groundwater. Many of them are indispensable to life but may be harmful at higher concentrations. Metals with toxic properties, which are among the most important inorganic contaminants of waters and soils, become hygienically serious. The presence of cadmium (Cd), mercury (Hg) and chromium (Cr) is currently one of the most recent risks. Toxic metals have a negative impact not only on the surrounding environment, but especially on human and animal health. They also have an impact on flora and fauna [3, 8, 15–17].

4. Pedospere

Soil is a natural formation that arises directly on the Earth's surface as a product of the interaction of climatic conditions, organisms, humans, relief and parent rocks Act 34/2014 Coll., amending and supplementing Act 220/2004 Coll., On the (Protection and Use of Agricultural Land). Soil is a complex system of abiotic and biotic components and is the result of soil-forming factors. It is created on the interface of the atmosphere, the lithosphere, the hydrosphere and the biosphere, which to a great extent influences its composition. In the soil-forming processes, abiotic and biotic environmental factors are applied together, and the result of their action is the abiotic-biotic component of the environment - soil. *The main abiotic factors* involved in soil formation include: parent (soil-forming) rock, relief, water and climatic conditions. The chemical composition of the soil depends primarily on the parent rock from which the soil originated, from the processes running in the soil and from the activity of man. Soil contains most oxygen (about 50%) and silicon (about 25%), other elements are mainly aluminum (clay), iron, calcium (limestone, gypsum), sodium, potassium, magnesium, hydrogen, titanium, in lesser amounts carbon, chlorine, phosphorus, sulfur and manganese. *Biotic agents* include soil edaphone. These factors are collectively called soil-forming factors. Edaphone is a living component of soil. It is a set of soil microorganisms, fungi, plants and animals. Soil organisms (geo bionti, edafonti) live in slots washed out by air or water, especially in the surface layers of the soil. For humification processes, plants, bacteria, and mycophytes are the most important. The root system of higher plants ensures the mechanical movement of the soil and keeps it loose. Bacteria break down organic matter in the soil. The soil contains both autotrophic and heterotrophic bacteria. Bacteria can have diverse functions in the soil. Decomposition of animal, plant and microbial residues is performed by heterotrophic bacteria. Chemoautotrophic bacteria in the soil are predominantly represented by nitrifying bacteria and, to a lesser extent, sulfur-oxidizing bacteria. The most common microbial cells in the soil are single-cell prokaryotes. Despite their high concentration in soil, fungal biomass predominates over the biomass of bacteria. Soil bacterial flora is extremely diverse and is dominated by Gram-positive bacteria. Fungi dominate the soil in terms of biomass amount. They are eukaryotic and have a mycelial morphology consisting of mycelia that surrounds the multinuclear cytoplasm. They live in symbiosis with most plant roots, which are of great importance for regulating nutrient uptake, aquatic connections and ultimately the growth of a plant partner in this community. Soil spore production allows to some extent their survival under unfavorable soil conditions. Fungi also include many important plant pathogens. Bacteria, worms, insects and other animals process plant residues in healthy soil. In this way, soil is enriched with substances that are vital for plants. However, if the soil is acidified by acid rain, the animals cannot live in it. Dead plant residues remain lying on the ground, no nutrients are created for the animals, and the food chain breaks. *Soil contamination, causes, monitoring*: we consider soil to be one of the main components of the Earth's ecosphere. It forms the basis of the nutritional chain at the end of which man stands [2, 18]. The most important soil characteristic is fertility, the ability of the soil to provide plants with water, air, nutrients in optimal quantities throughout the vegetation [19]. The soil system is a very specific component and to some extent can effectively and naturally eliminate various foreign substances. Soil and ecosystem components - water and air - are basic indicators of pollution. The soil loses most due to contamination since its ability to eliminate the negative effects caused by the natural and anthropogenic activity of man become limited [20–22]. Major problem of consumer society is waste production. The issue of waste does not end with the disposal of waste in landfills. Precipitation waters that infiltrate through landfills are contaminated with waste materials. Such landfill leachates can then contaminate the soil or the bedrock where the landfill is located. Another factor that negatively affects soil environmental functions is the contamination of soil by water and air. Pollutants in air and water are mainly from industrial production. *Toxic heavy metals*, like biogenic metals, are present in the soil in two mobilities. They occur in the liquid phase as hydrated ions or as soluble organic and inorganic complexes. In the solid phase they are in the form of insoluble precipitates on the surface of organic and inorganic colloids in exchangeable and specifically absorbed form. A dynamic equilibrium is created between the various forms, in accordance with the characteristics of the system. If e.g., a large amount of toxic substance gets into the soil, absorption and precipitation reactions predominate. On the other hand, when the acidity of the soil increases, the number of mobile forms increases, i.e., the concentration of metal ions in solution increases. Contamination of the soil by sulfur dioxide exhales is leads to its *acidification*. Low pH causes increased mobility of cadmium and aluminum, which can intoxicate plants. Other contaminants also enter the soil through sedimentation: nitrogen oxides, lead, cadmium, arsenic, fly ash, chromium, nickel, organic compounds. Lead polluting soil comes mainly from automobile traffic. The source of cadmium is the burning of fossil fuels. The arsenic from the power plant ash dissolves well in the water and therefore does not accumulate in the topsoil but passes into the lower layers. Acidification of the soil in already contaminated areas is particularly dangerous as heavy metal compounds are normally insoluble, but when mobilized, they can result in a serious environmental damage (*timed chemical bomb*). Soil is an important geochemical reservoir, which relatively easily accumulates heavy metals. They are removed only very slowly, by leaching processes into subsurface waters or by plant bioaccumulation. Soil is the starting point for the entry of risky elements into crops and through forage into animal products [23, 24]. Soil contamination with water occurs as a result of soil irrigation or rainfall activity. Erosion is one of the most serious problems threatening soil worldwide. The erosion is due to the spread of mountain farming, the excavation of forests, the deterioration of the soil's water regime, the plowing of grasslands, the artificial regulation of watercourses, the wrong land cultivation. The result of erosion is the drainage of soil parts, humus, nutrients, crop reduction. As reported by the authors [13, 15, 25, 26]. industrial emissions primarily affect the pollution of agricultural and forest land. Especially increased content of lead (Pb), zinc (Zn), tin (Sn), cadmium (Cd), aluminum (Al), copper (Cu), nickel (Ni), mercury (Hg), manganese (Mn), and arsenic (As) was found in the vicinity of metallurgical factories. All metals usually get into the soil, but increasingly those components that dominate the immission type. The most important metal pollutants of soil are mercury (Hg), cadmium (Cd) and lead (Pb), which are generally toxic to humans and animals [2, 3, 9, 16, 27].

4.1 Health risks of environmental pollution, risk analysis, evaluation

Increasingly polluted environment, preservatives, dyes and flavorings present in the food are heavily burdening the body. Pesticides for weed control, chemical fertilizers, and nitrates can be carcinogenic when getting into organism. Automobile exhaust gases, ozone, formaldehyde, wood disinfectants and preservatives, insecticides, paint solvents and the like contaminate air, damage the respiratory tract and weaken the immune system [26]. This is why methods for assessing health risks (e.g. questionnaires, risk assessment, analyses, diagrams, use of geographic information systems) are extremely important. *Risk Analysis* - [28] states that it is very important to determine the level of danger to human health and animals in a given location and at the same time to take account of future use of a respective area. In general, the principles of the health risk assessment, hazard determination and hazard identification, (evaluation of dose - response relationship, exposure evaluation & assessment, risk characterization are applied). In assessing the health risks and adverse effects of metals, it is important to evaluate not only their presence and overall concentration in the environment and in food, but also their chemical and mineral forms that affect their persistence and bioavailability. The effects of sudden metal uptake into organisms may have the character of *"acute disease"*. Metals, with regard to the accumulation in target organs of the organism, cause disease manifestations after periods with different length (weeks to years) and the clinical picture has the character of "*chronic disease*" [11, 29]. *The aim of the assessment* is to determine the harmfulness of chemicals or other risk factors occurring on the site and to assess whether the substance or risk factor has the ability to damage the body. In general, this part of the risk assessment process describes the quantitative relationship between dose and extent of adverse effect (injury, disease, death). This step requires two basic types of extrapolation using different mathematical models. These are extrapolations - interspecific (experimental animal - human) and extrapolation to the low dose area [10]. At present, the *protection* of *environment* is seen as a necessary condition for the existence and further development of human society. It includes activities to prevent pollution or damage to the environment, respectively for the reduction and/or elimination of pollution. It is either general protection (air, soil, water), special protection (protected areas, plants, animals,) or the protection of cultural monuments. *The creation of the environment* is understood as a purposeful human activity that is organized on a scientific basis, aiming at optimizing the natural and artificial components of the landscape. *The aim of environmental care* is to maintain or improve its quality with respect to all organisms, while respecting all principles of sustainable living. This environmental care is called environmentalism [7, 13, 30].

4.2 Heavy metals and their importance in environmental pollution, sources, form

Heavy metals are among the common environmental pollutants resulting from both industrial and agricultural production [31]. They are not subject to biological degradation, and their levels are gradually increasing in the individual environmental components: water, air, foodstuffs [29, 32]. They are released into the environment from natural sources (weathering) and by erosion of some minerals and rocks. As stated by [33] the natural increased incidence of heavy metals and other risk elements is mainly in the areas of geochemical anomalies. Regarding pesticides (containing heavy metals), their use has been suspended and is no longer the source of this type of pollution. Metal production (their heat treatment), chemical, engineering, energy production, fossil fuel combustion, waste, food production flushing, fertilization, etc. are among the major *anthropogenic sources* of environmental pollution. As [34] report, metallurgy of ferrous and non-ferrous ores (the impact of non-ferrous ore metallurgy is predominant in mercury) contributes most to emissions of mercury (Hg), cadmium (Cd), lead (Pb), chromium (Cr), copper (Cu) and zinc (Zn). Combustion of fossil fuels contributes significantly to the emissions of most heavy metals, glass production is a significant source of lead (Pb) and cadmium (Cd) emissions, and transport, despite the dynamic increase in the use of unleaded petrol, complements these sources. In the past, alkyl lead compounds (tetra-ethyl lead) were used as anti-knock additives in gasoline, thereby increasing the concentration of lead in the air. Thus, pollutants are introduced into the environment from various sources and based on their physico-chemical properties. They are transported and participate in biochemical cycles in individual environmental components (air, water, soil, rocks, segments). [35] states that heavy metals constitute one of the most dangerous groups of pollutants. Their amount in the environment is given by content, quantity and movement in all spheres of the environment. The side effects of heavy metal emissions are dangerous, they usually get into the environment (the air) in an uncontrolled way. In the environment, they can occur as simple complexes with inorganic ligands (in the aqueous environment, the form of the metal is affected by physico-chemical properties: pH, temperature, ionic strength), as chelates with organic ligands (sorbed to solid surfaces), free metals. In the terrestrial environment, fate, bioavailability and mobility of metals are influenced by: soil type, oxidation–reduction processes and cationic solid phase capacity [36]. More detailed information on the specific effects of individual heavy metals on cells, tissues, and organs of animals is obtained and validated within laboratory animal experiments. However, the results of the experimental application cannot be considered generally valid. Mostly, the experiment only works with the substance being studied individually, which does not occur alone in the environment. All animal species may not respond to the toxic substance in the same way. In the response of the organism to the action of a toxic substance, the overall momentary state of the organism, its life phase and gender are important. Taking all these factors into account during an experiment is almost impossible. Therefore, despite the systematic research, there is still some concern over formulating the environmental and hazardous concentrations of these substances. However, these doubts do not justify the presence of heavy metals in the environment being taken lightly or underestimated. The combination of overexploitation of natural resources, coercive forced population growth and economic developments, as well as a lack of government regulations can increase the flow of toxic metals into the environment in all countries. By 2010, a significant increase in emissions of mercury (Hg), cadmium (Cd), copper (Cu) and a decrease in lead (Pb) emissions and deposition was expected in Europe [2]. Heavy metals cause a wide range of toxic biochemical effects and thus adversely affect organs and systems in humans and animals [37, 38]. Therefore, they pose a serious risk to health regardless of the source from which they enter the body. Some heavy metals (e.g., manganese, copper, zinc) are needed for physiological processes, but other toxic heavy metals (especially cadmium, mercury, lead) are environmental pollutants [39] and do not have any known physiological roles. Conversely, they may adversely affect health [40] and thus induce a variety of adverse effects including reproductive disorders [41] nutritional deficiencies, endocrine disorders [42, 43] or immunodeficiency disorders; they can induce tumor formation and other health-damaging chronic conditions [32, 44]. Currently, there is also a strong focus on low-dose exposures (environmentally relevant concentrations) of these metals that may affect human and animal reproductive health [3, 45, 46]. Ecologists and environmentalists duly address this issue and take into account the contexts that have not yet been considered. Even if the concentrations of heavy metals with regard to the health safety of living organisms are limited within the monitored areas, environmentalists are the ones drawing attention to many natural processes that cause the concentration of toxic elements to become a real danger. Certain metals are needed for normal body function. They are part of the enzymes and take different roles in metabolic processes and electron transfer - manganese (Mn), copper (Cu), nickel (Ni), molybdenum (Mo), cobalt (Co), iron (Fe), zinc (Zn), however, at higher concentrations they can already become toxic. Heavy metals are characterized by varying degrees of toxicity and different effects on living organisms. The subject of world monitoring is strongly toxic elements - mercury (Hg), cadmium (Cd), lead (Pb), arsenic (As), which have almost no purpose in the organism [47]. Metals are found bound in various inorganic compounds, but can also enter complex organic systems. They are persistent, non-degradable, biologically active with high bioaccumulation potential. They form a natural part of the Earth's surface composition and therefore occur everywhere in various concentrations. The natural balance of elements is also impaired by human activity. Together with the development of modern technology, production and consumption of metals and metalloids are growing rapidly, too. This is particularly true for non-ferrous metals, some of which have until recently been produced in incomparably lower amounts (e.g. laboratory scale) - beryllium (Be), titanium (Tl) gallium (Ga), selenium (Se), molybdenum (Mo), wolfram (W). Also, the production of classic colored metals which are gradually finding new types of applications, is increasing,. This is especially true for aluminum (Al), lead (Pb), nickel (Ni), chromium (Cr), antimony (Sb), mercury (Hg). Increasing the concentration of the above metals in the environment - air, water, soil and foodstuffs, is a serious hygiene problem and its scale is still becoming larger [23, 34, 48–50]. In general, metals are highly reactive elements which, on the one hand, are essential (they are components of some enzymes), on the other hand they are capable of damaging different enzymes or interfering with different levels of signal transduction processes in cells.

4.3 Heavy metals and food chain

There is a comprehensive versatile and complex network of food chains in nature. They are interconnected, while the function of the individual elements of the food chains may vary. This causes the symbiotic organism to become dysbiotic, useful changes to harmful, or pathogenic [51]. The common population is also contaminated with the food chain [52] since it has a major impact on human (but also animal) nutrition, lifestyle and life expressions. Animals are much more exposed to the impact of the geochemical environment than humans, as they serve as effective buffers in the nutritional chain, in reducing the adverse effects of the environment on the consumer. According to [53] optimizing the animal nutrition can affect the human food chain. Most heavy metals get into the organism by plant or animal food (the load from air or drinking water is significantly lower). They are converted either into harmless metabolites (detoxification) that are easily excreted, or harmful, reactive products are formed. [54] states that the increased content of especially cadmium (Cd), mercury (Hg), chromium (Cr), arsenic (As), lead (Pb) and nickel (Ni) in agricultural soils may pose a potential risk of contamination of agricultural production. In most countries, including, the applicable legislation determines the maximum permissible concentrations (MPCs) for individual heavy metals (drinking water, air, foodstuffs of plant or animal origin). Therefore, the protection of the food chain from heavy metal contamination, and its follow-up checks are considered to be important in terms of health security. As reported by [55] food safety is a set of measures (animal health and welfare section, food and feed sector) and with their implementation, the safety of all components within the food chain is ensured. According to [56] the occurrence of contaminants in environmental components and in agricultural and food production is monitored through random check-ups and regular monitoring. The relationship between animal health, human health and the environment has been known for a long time. Potential contaminants and their total amount for both veterinary and public health are broad and vary according to their source, chemical nature and mechanism of action on biological systems. [57] state that the prevention of human and animal health from chemical risks implies their control throughout the food chain - field-table. Food quality control with the participation of state health surveillance in the Slovak Republic is one of the essential tasks of food surveillance and the limits of foreign substances in food commodities are harmonized in accordance with the limits of the European Union [58–61].

4.4 Impact of selected heavy metals-Hg and Cd on humans, animals and the environment

The transport of heavy metals in the atmosphere and their subsequent deposition depends on the following factors: the form in which the metal is found to escape into the atmosphere (solid or gaseous phase), their chemical reaction in the atmosphere, the height and location of the point source of emission, local geographic conditions, speed and direction of wind, rain washing and other meteorological requirements [12]. Pollution of the environment is now a global phenomenon, not excluding the territory of Slovakia and contributes to the deterioration of living and working conditions [2]. Recently, great attention has been paid to the impact of toxic heavy metals and their compounds (especially mercury, cadmium, lead) on human and animal health, which are considered to be dangerous and non-degradable contaminants in the environment. However, a suitable marker for early diagnosis of heavy metal exposure (including drinking water sources) has not yet been developed, which is perceived as a relatively serious problem [62].

As reported by several authors [44, 63, 64] the main consequence of the negative effect of environmental contaminants is the disruption of the optimal immune reactivity of the organism, the occurrence of allergies, increased susceptibility to pathogenic agents, higher occurrence of tumors, affecting reproduction. History shows us a number of global industrial accidents pointing to the negative effects. An important part in creating a good living environment for both humans and livestock is active health creation. It is based on two fundamental phenomena. It is a principle of complexity of measures, respecting variability of the effects of relationships and factors - the internal and external environment of the organism [7].

4.5 Cadmium - sources of cadmium in the environment, the effects of its occurrence

The main sources of cadmium include volcanic activity, weathering of rocks, or forest fires [65]. It gets into the environment by mining and processing of fossil fuels, ferrous and non-ferrous ores, limestone, in cement production [66]. It can be found in Cd-Ni batteries, stabilizers of plastics, home appliances. Cadmium also occurs in synthetic superphosphate and in naturally occurring superphosphates. Cadmium (yellow-orange) paints are added to coatings, gums, textiles, glass and ceramics. Along with zinc (Zn), it occurs in ores and soil at a ratio of 1:100 to 1:1000. It is usually found in the form of cadmium sulfide (CdS) in ores which also contain lead (Pb), zinc (Zn) and copper (Cu). Unlike mercury, it is not subject to biotransformation and cannot be released as an alkyl derivative from the organism. It is now widely used for its anticorrosive effects and serves as a base for electroplating and nickel plating. It is also widely used in making jewelry. It can enter the atmosphere due to poor waste incineration technology (higher cadmium exposure is near the smelter where ores blended with Cd are melted) or oil products [67]. According to WHO, the largest part of cadmium is bound to fine particles (<1 μm) in air, which can then spread up to 1–2 km. Thus, cadmium builds up in soil, water and then enters the food chain. In soil and in some plants, accumula tion occurs especially at low soil pH (e.g. leaves, rice). In agricultural soils, the accumulation of cadmium may be associated with the application of (phosphate fertilizers, sewage sludge, some fungicides [66, 68, 69].). The concentration of cadmium in the soil ranges from 0.01 to 0.7 $mg.kg^{-1}$ and is most cumulative in the 0–5 cm layer. With increasing depth there is a decrease in its concentration. In the process of weathering rocks (content not exceeding 0.3 $mg.kg^{-1}$), it is easily transformed into a solution and its occurrence is in the form of Cd^{2+}. According to [70], cadmium intake by plants increases with the presence of chlorine in the soil and the content is also significantly affected by soil microorganisms. The way of farming, the time of harvesting the crop and also the environment (climate) affects the cadmium transfer into the plants. This suggests that increased cadmium content in soil is the result of increased cadmium absorption by plants, but, as [71] states, the bioavailability of cadmium also depends on soil solution composition, soil pH, and redox potential. Soil has the ability to somewhat eliminate the negative effects of pollution [22]. Compared to other environmental components, soil status is exceptional. Air and water may move (dilution occurs), and if the source of pollution ceases to be active, there is also a limitation or total elimination of pollution. However, in case of soil contamination by risk elements, we have to realize that this is an irreversible process, it cannot be observed immediately and therefore it is all the more serious. In waters, cadmium accompanies zinc at substantially lower concentrations. According to the higher cadmium content (Cd) has been repeatedly detected in water flowing right by zinc mines. The solubility in water is determined by the solubility of $CdCO_3$ and Cd $(OH)_2$. It is generally presumed that people (but also animals) are the most sensitive cadmium intake group when environment is concerned. The main source of cadmium intake for humans and animals is food, feed and beverages. It is estimated that the average daily dietary intake of cadmium is 50 μg. Up to 25% of the daily intake is retained in the body. The content in dairy products is higher. The lethal dose for oral intake is 350–8900 μg [11].

The impact of the toxic effects of cadmium on the organism: Relative the toxic effect, cadmium is one of the elements that is of great concern for its toxicity and widespread environmental impact. In humans, the main source of Cd exposure is food [72] and the bioavailability of cadmium from food is an important determinant of its potential risk. Cadmium is one of the 10 most toxic substances for human and animal health [39, 73]. Cigarette smoking is also an important source of cadmium accumulation in the body. As reported by author [37] cadmium can cause functional and morphological changes in organs and tissues, and is also strongly neurotoxic. When the exposure to cadmium in environmental components is short term, there may be no health consequences, but from the perspective of long-term exposure (individuals who are more sensitive to toxic effects - infants and children) certain symptoms may occur [70]. The detoxification of the organism is slow (cadmium is characterized by a high accumulation coefficient) and there is a danger of chronic intoxication. Chemically, cadmium is very similar to zinc (it is a part of food), it has an important role for the proper development and health of the organism. However, the similar chemical form of these elements can cause problems as cadmium easily enters various enzymatic reactions instead of zinc, and biochemical processes take place in a different way (e.g., blocking the insulin cycle) and serious health complications occur [3, 74]. Cadmium gets into the organism in three ways: by inhalation, gastrointestinal tract and absorption through the skin. According to WHO, 50–2600 tons of cadmium are emitted annually from natural resources. The atmosphere is polluted by 3300–12,500 tons annually through human activity. In order to eliminate the negative effect on the living organism, [75] recommends a concentration of 5 $ng.m^{-3}$ as a non-carcinogenic cadmium limit in the air. Current levels in rural areas usually do not exceed 0.4 $ng.m^{-3}$, and in cities they range from 0.2 to 2.5 $ng.m^{-3}$. According to in the vicinity of certain industrial agglomerations, this concentration can be significantly higher. WHO has determined a provisional tolerable weekly intake (PTWI) for cadmium at 7 $\mu g.kg^{-1}$ of body weight. Since food is a major source of cadmium for most of the population, attention has also been paid to its quality as well as to the reduction of cadmium contamination of the environment. With an average absorption of about 5% of the amount received, about 0.5–1 μg of cadmium is retained daily in the organism. Based on epidemiological studies, there has been an increase in lung cancer and prostate cancer in long-term cadmium inhalation. In hazardous operations, inhalation intake is currently strictly controlled. The human lethal dose is 0.3–8.9 g. IARC [100] (International Agency for Research on Cancer) classifies Cd as the first category carcinogen for humans and animals.

4.6 Mercury - sources of mercury in the environment, the effects of mercury

Mercury is commonly found in the natural environment as it is a part of the Earth's crust. Its origin can be geogenic and anthropogenic. Mercury gets into the environment during its production and processing of products (production of electrodes, electrical equipment, dyes, measuring and control equipment, use in dentistry, chemical laboratories, etc.). In a year, this is estimated at 10,000–30,000 tons of mercury; and it gets into the environment by evaporating from the surface of the Earth and the oceans (vapor of metallic mercury, volatile organic compounds), [48]. The conversion of mercury (present in the form of ions) in a volatile form can theoretically occur in three ways: by chemical reaction to elemental mercury (not previously found in nature), by reduction to elemental mercury by microorganisms, plants, animals, and by biotransformation to more volatile organo-mercury compounds (alkyl compounds), [76]. According to the most recent data, 5207 × 10^6 g of mercury is released from the natural sources annually into the atmosphere, and 2909 × 10^6 g (total 8116 × 10^6 g) of mercury from anthropogenic sources. The main anthropogenic sources by which mercury enters the atmosphere is the combustion of fossil fuels (1422 × 10^6 g.year^{-1}), gold mining (400 × 10^6 g. year^{-1}), waste management (187 × 10^6 g.year^{-1}), production of non-ferrous metals (310 × 10^6 g.year^{-1}), cement production (236 × 10^6 g.year^{-1}) [34, 77]. Global mercury emissions from natural resources are estimated at 3.0 × 10^6 g.year^{-1}. The average mercury (Hg) content in the Earth's crust is about 0.067 ppm. *Air, water, soil* - elemental mercury vapors released from the Earth's crust rise to the atmosphere (amount of about 18 mg.m^{-3}), where they are oxidized to divalent mercury and from there the compounds get into the water reservoirs by rain. Divalent mercury in the sediments at the bottom of the seas and lakes is methylated to methyl mercury by the action of microorganisms. It enters the food chain - phytoplankton - zooplankton - small fish - big fish. At the top of this chain are animals (that feed on fish), including humans. Within this chain, the process of bioaccumulation of ethylmercury occurs. As reported by [11, 78], its concentration is gradually increasing, with the values at the top of the chain about a million times higher than the concentration of methylmercury in the surrounding water. In general, large and longer-living fish (shark, tuna, mackerel, pike) also contain more mercury [48, 79, 80]. Under "European Commission Decision 93/351", the value of Hg in the meat of fish living in relatively uncontaminated areas should be below 0.5 gg^{-1}.The concentration of mercury in the air ranges from 1 to 5 mg.m^{-3} in rural areas and 7–10 mg.m^{-3} in cities. The enrichment of soils with mercury is caused by the burning of coal, the occurrence of cinnabar deposits, but also by applying mercury-based fungicides. The use of sewage and urban sludge and fertilizers is also a source of mercury soil pollution. However, this is not just about soil contamination, but also about secondary effect on vegetation growing on it [81]. Mercury gets into the soil in the range of 0.02–03 mg.kg^{-1}. The concentration of mercury in uncontaminated soils should be within the range of 0.02–0.2 mg.kg^{-1} [82]. Average concentrations affected by human activity are in the range of 0.1–0.4 mg.kg^{-1}, and in the vicinity of industrial enterprises and crematoria up to 1.8 mg.kg^{-1}, in the third of Slovakia's territory the content of total mercury is higher in woody plants (the value exceeds 0.12 mg.kg^{-1}) [11, 83, 84]. The natural content in the soil is from several, up to tens of μg.kg^{-1}. The use of mercury and its compounds has spread rapidly, and this fact cannot remain without consequences for: the environment, living organisms, including humans and animals. Therefore it is important to create favorable living conditions also for livestock (active health creation) based on the fundamental phenomena - complexity of measures and respect for the variability of the effects of relationships and factors between the internal and external environment [7]. **Effects of toxic action of mercury on the organism:** Regarding the effects of toxic effects on the organism, mercury is given a relatively high attention. Its toxicity depends on the physical properties of the individual forms. However, there are differences among them, based on the way of exposure, the metabolism itself, the way of excretion. It is known that the more mobile the form of mercury is, the more toxic it becomes. These properties are due to the structure of the molecule (e.g., behavior in biosystems, stability, excretion rates, etc.) [49, 85]. The negative impact not only on the health of people but also on the health and the performance of the animals results from an increased incidence of mercury, especially in polluted areas. The hygienic quality of animal products is lower, the content of toxic elements in meat and dairy products is higher and the reproductive and growth indicators get reduced [9, 86]. Mercury is the world's only liquid metal that gets into the body most often by inhalation of mercury vapor, and up to 80% of these is absorbed in the lungs. The absorption of elemental mercury in the GIT is very low, less than 1%. [87] report that compounds containing divalent mercury are absorbed in GIT more, even up to 10%. Further, it is taken into consideration that oral administration may be accidental, or in contact with skin. As stated by [88], this metal has a high affinity for phosphates, cysteine and histidinyl side chains of proteins, but also for purines, porphyrins and pteridines. Mercury, along with its compounds, is one of the high-toxic poisons (5 times more toxic than lead). The harmful daily human dose is 0.4 mg, the lethal dose is 150–300 mg. The condition of its toxic effect is the oxidation of Hg^0 to Hg^{1+} up to Hg^{2+}. After oxidation, Hg^{2+} binds to -SH groups of proteins, which are thereby inactivated. Upon absorption, a large proportion of mercury (depending on the type of compound and the site of absorption) gets into circulation. A part enters the erythrocytes and another part binds to the ligands in the plasma. The ratio of mercury content in plasma and in erythrocytes is about 1: 1. In erythrocytes, mercury (Hg) binds to the -SH group of hemoglobin. Elemental mercury (e.g. in mercury vapor poisoning) is oxidized to divalent cation. In plasma, mercury binds to albumin and other plasma proteins that contain free -SH groups. Exposure to mercury increases the amount of metallothionein (low molecular weight protein), which to some extent prevents kidney damage [11, 89, 90]. Elemental mercury and some of its organic compounds easily cross membranes (e.g., the erythrocyte membrane) and, unlike some other heavy metals (e.g. cadmium), easily cross the placental blood–brain barrier, too. In the complex with glutathione it is excreted in the bile, but it also reaches the sweat, salivary and dairy glands. In humans, the mean half-life of excretion for inorganic mercury is 60 days, for alkyl compounds of mercury 70 days [73]. The kidneys are the site of the greatest accumulation of mercury and also the major site of its excretion. There are several hypotheses explaining the mechanism of mercury excretion in the kidneys. One of them is the hypothesis that part of it gets into the urine in binding to albumin and then is reabsorbed (by endocytosis) in the proximal tubule. Another part is excreted in binding to glutathione, which is, similar to bile, hydrolyzed to amino acids by γ-glutamyltransferase and dipeptidases, and such amino acids are then reabsorbed by the Na-dependent transport system [91]. Mercury is excreted in the feces and urine. For inorganic mercury, the excretion half-life (both acute and chronic) is 1–3 months, for methylmercury it is 50 days. Since methylmercury permeates the hair, the level is used as a marker of mercury exposure [11, 92]. Food that has been contaminated with methylmercury (especially fish) are among the most common sources of exposure to organic mercury. At the end of the 19th century, [93] described the so-called pink disease (acrodynia - sporadic and predominant pediatric syndrome associated with calomel in toothpaste and other forms of inorganic mercury) related to an allergic reaction in hypersensitive people. Abnormal reddening of the skin has occurred, as well as peeling of the skin (area of the hands, legs, feet), pain threshold reduction, swelling. Acrodynia has been found in infants but also in older children who have used diapers treated with phenylmercury (an organic form of mercury). In spite of the scientifically-based study, mercury is still a part of various cosmetics and pharmaceutical compositions. However, it should be noted that the skin reactions to mercury are relatively rare, even scarce. The concentration of mercury in the blood in the general population (the result of dietary intake) is mainly in the form of organic compounds, but it is present in the urine mainly in inorganic form. Why this is the case (difference in form) yet needs to be further explored in mammals. As reported by [94], mercury concentration in blood increases with fish consumption. However, larger areas of amalgam fillers, which may be the source of increased urinary excretion, also need to be considered. Other so-called immunotoxic responses can also be induced when exposed to inorganic mercury - Kawasaki disease, rash, cracking of the lips, fever, photophobia, pharyngitis, peeling of the skin on the palms of the hands and feet, tachycardia, affection of the lymphatic tissue - these are symptoms afflicted by sufferers. Urine levels of mercury have been shown to be higher in the affected patients. [93] reports that infants but also older children have more sensitive organisms than adults, and that explains the higher absorption of inorganic mercury. Among the organic mercury compounds, thiomersal (thimerosal, mertiolate, sodium ethylmercurithiosalicylate) is known as being used as a preservative in childhood vaccination since the 1930s. The thiomersal composition is 49.6 wt% Hg - it is metabolized to EtHg and thiosalicylate. The vaccine dose for children contains about 2.5 mg Hg in 0.5 ml. [95, 96] have expressed concern that the developing CNS could be harmed in children in the first half year of life. Possible health consequences: delayed speech development, impaired concentration, local hypersensitive responses, the spectrum of autism disorders. With long term administration of gamma globulin (containing thiomersal), acrodynia has occasionally been confirmed. Based on these findings, thiomersal was requested to be removed from vaccines. However, it continues to be used in some countries to these days. According to [97] at high doses of EtHg the undesirable effects are similar to high doses of MeHg. However, the effect of low dose of EtHg remains unclear, more recent data [98] describe EtHg to be less neurotoxic than MeHg. The effects of mercury on health depend on several factors (form, dose, duration of exposure). International organizations Health Care Without Harm and the Health & Environment Alliance advocate accelerated reduction of environmental pollution by mercury in the European Union as well as worldwide and raise awareness of its destructive impact on the human fetal brain (arises during the early development of the fetus by methylmercury). It has a damaging effect on the development of the nervous system, and such damage is mostly irreversible. [99] states that the source of intense interest in the scientific community is primarily three chemical forms as a source of exposure: methyl mercury in fish, mercury vapor from amalgam dental fillings, and ethyl mercury in vaccines. US EPA (Environmental Protection Agency) classifies inorganic mercury into Group D "substances that do not have carcinogenic effects on humans" but [100] is considering reviewing the inclusion of inorganic mercury according to EPA. Organic forms of mercury - methyl mercury and its compounds are, according to IARC, rated as possible carcinogens [63].

5. Conclusion

Population health, as a universal value and primary human rights, is a fundamental economic resource not only for the individual but also for the whole of society. One of the main starting points for solving the relationship between man and the environment is the planned nature protection. The environment is everything that creates natural conditions for the existence of organisms, including humans, and is a prerequisite for their further development. The work was supported by VEGA 2/0125/17.

Author details

Iveta Cimboláková[1]*, Ivan Uher[1], Katarína Veszelits Laktičová[2], Mária Vargová[2], Tatiana Kimáková[1] and Ingrid Papajová[3]

1 Pavol Jozef Šafarik University, Kosice, Slovak Republic

2 University of Veterinary Medicine and Pharmacy in Kosice, Kosice, Slovak Republic

3 Slovak Academy of Science, Department of Environmental and Plant Parasitology, Kosice, Slovak Republic

*Address all correspondence to: iveta.cimbolakova@upjs.sk

References

[1] Kontrišová O. Základné princípy bioindikácie a biomonitoringu životného prostredia. Životné Prostredie. 2006;**40**(2):61-64

[2] Fargašová A. Environmentálna toxikológia a všeobecná toxikológia. Distribúcia kovov v životnom prostredí. UK Bratislava: PF; 2009. pp. 1-25. ISBN 9788096967568

[3] Cimboláková I. Vplyv rizikových prvkov na zdravie zvierat a životné prostredie: dizertačná práca. Košice; 2013. 111 p. CD-ROM

[4] Hothorn LA. Selected biostatistical aspects of the validation of in vitro toxicological assays. ATLA. 2002;**30**:93-98

[5] Lieskovská Z, Palúchová K. Možnosti implementácie princípov hodnotenia zdravotných rizík do procesu EIA. In: Zborník Medzinárodný workshop o posudzovaní vplyvov na životné prostredie. 2003. pp. 47-55. ISBN 80-8069-246-7

[6] Noskovič J. Tvorba a ochrana životného prostredia. Nitra: SPU; 2003. 141 p. ISBN 80-8069-578-4

[7] Ondrašovičová O. Zdravie a tvorba životných podmienok zvierat. Ekológia a veterinárna medicína VIII. Košice: UVLF; 2011. p. 7. ISBN 978-80-8077-249-9

[8] Iveta C, Silvia FI, et al. Výskum v medicíne a etika. 1st ed. Košice: Equilibria; 2015. 65 p. ISBN 9788081522949

[9] Tatiana K. Ortuť v životnom prostredí ako rizikový faktor zdravia/ Tatiana Kimáková; recenzenti Kamila Bernasovská, Janka Poráčová. 1st ed. Košice: Univerzita Pavla Jozefa Šafárika v Košiciach; 2017. 148 p. ISBN 9788081524783

[10] Tatiana K, Iveta C, Silvia FI, Miroslava D, Nikita B. Environment a jeho etické aspekty. In: Kimáková T et al., editors. recenzenti Ľubomír Straka, Bernasovská Kamila. 1st ed. Košice: Univerzita Pavla Jozefa Šafárika v Košiciach; 2015. 88 p. ISBN 9788081522963

[11] Buchancová J. Pracovné lekárstvo a toxikológia. Osveta: Martin; 2003. 1095 p. ISBN 80-8063-113-1

[12] Jandačka J, Malcho M, Mikulík M. Ekologické aspekty zámeny fosílnych palív za biomasu. INTERREG IIIA SR-ČR 2004-2006; 2008. 226 p. ISBN: 978-80-969595-5-6

[13] Ondrašovič M, Kol A. Ochrana životného prostredia a verejného zdravia. Košice; Vydavateľstvo UVLF Košice, SR, väzba brožovaná. 2013. 271 p

[14] Veszelits Laktičová K, Čisláková L, Vargová M, Hromada R, Ondrašovič M, Chvojka D, et al. Hygiena zdravotníckych a farmaceutických zariadení. Košice; Vydavateľstvo UVLF Košice, SR. 2016. ISBN 978-80-8077-495-0

[15] Lahučký L, Árway J, Bystrická J, Čéry J. Obsah ťažkých kovov v poľnohospodárskej produkcii dopestovanej v metalicky zaťaženom regióne Slovenska. Agriculture. 2009;**55**(3):156-163

[16] Cimboláková I, Nováková J, Lovásová E. Ťažké kovy-ich vplyv na životné prostredie, potravinový reťazec a zdravie. In: Situácia v ekologicky zaťažených regiónoch Slovenska a strednej Európy XVIII. vedecké sympózium s medzinárodnou účasťou: Hrádok 22-23. Košice; Slovenská banícka spoločnosť ZSVTS, c2009, Signatura: 273665. 2009. pp. 17-20. ISBN 9788097003418

[17] Korineková M, Havlík T. Odstraňovanie ťažkých kovov z roztokov sorpciou na zeolit. Acta Metallurgica Slovaca. 2006;**12**(49):208-213

[18] Štyriak I, Szabová T, Alačová A, Koščová M, Štyriaková I. Vplyv ťažkých kovov na pôdnu mikroflóru. Acta Montanistica Slovaca. 2002;**7**(4): 271-273

[19] Ništiar F, Lukačínová A, Rácz O, Beňačka R. Celoživotná expozícia nízkymi dávkami ťažkých kovov počas troch generácií u potkanov. Úskalia a východiská. In: Beňačka R, editor. Patofyziológia 2010. Zborník prác. Košice: UPJŠ LF; 2010. pp. 53-58. ISBN 978-80-7097-827-6

[20] Čéry J, Árvay J, Stanovič R. Monitoring hygieny poľnohospodárskej pôdy v regióne Brekov, 8. Vedecká konferencia doktorandov a ml. vedeckých pracovníkov. Nitra: FPV UKF; 2007. pp. 455-460

[21] Dercová K, Makovníková J, Barančíková G, Žuffa J. Bioremediácia toxických kovov kontaminujúcich vody a pôdy. Chemicke Listy. 2005;**99**:682-693

[22] Mikuška R, Muchová Z. Kvalita dlhodobo skladovanej potravinárskej pšenice z pohľadu kontaminácie ťažkými kovmi. Nitra: Rizikové factory potravového reťazca V., SPU; 2005. pp. 230-234. ISBN 80-8069-593-8

[23] Fabián G, Priesol J. Základy environmentálnej chémie, UMB Banská bystrica. Banská Bystrica: Fakulta prírodných vied; 2009. 112 p. ISBN - 9788080837310

[24] Stanovič R, Árvay J, Melicháčová S, Szabóová G, Peltznerová L. Obsah kadmia, olova a medi na pozemku v intenzávne poľnohospodársky využívanej oblasti južného Slovenska. Acta fytotechnica et zootechnica. 2009:618-626

[25] Abas ANYMJ, Rahman MRB, Tahir NA, Rushdi NM, Simoneit BRT. Levels and distributions of organic source tracers in air and roadside dust particles of Kuala Lumpur, Malaysia. Environmental Geology. 2007;**52**(8):1485-1500

[26] Slávik M. Nekvalita života a jej vplyv na naše zdravie. In: Psychosociálne a zdravotné aspekty nekvality života. Zborník príspevkov z vedeckej konferencie s medzinárodnou účasťou, Prešov. 2006. pp. 101-105. ISBN 978-80-8068-927-8

[27] Bujnovský R. Analýza príčin degradácie pôdy ako predpoklad trvalo udržateľného využívania tohto prírodného zdroja. In: I. ročník medzinárodnej konferencie Zem v pasci? Analýza zložiek životného prostredia, Krpáčovo, 2006, s.1, An update. Electrophoresis. Vol. 30. 2009. pp. 92-99. ISBN 80-228-1553-1555

[28] Semple S. Assessing occupational and environmental exposure. Occupational Medicine. 2005;**55**:419-424

[29] Legáth J. Ochrana životného prostredia metódou odhadu rizika chemických látok pre jednotlivé zložky ekosystému. In: Beseda et al., editors. Aktuálne problémy kontaminácie životného prostredia z hľadiska toxikológie a ekotoxikológie. Zvolen: Fakulta ekológie a environmentalistiky, Technická univerzita; 2000. pp. 6-13. ISBN 80-228-0980-2

[30] Ondrašovičová O, Ondrašovič M, Sasáková N. Veterinárna starostlivosť o životné prostredie. 1st ed. Košice: Edičné stredisko UVL; 2009. 247 p. ISBN 978-80-8077-174-4

[31] Tipping E, Lawror AJ, Lofts S, Shotbolt L. Simulating the long-term chemistry of an upland UK catchment: Heavy metals. Environmental Pollution. 2006;**141**:139-150

[32] Lukačinová A, Beňačka R, Lovásová E, Rácz O, Ništiar F. Reproduction parameters in low dose chronic exposure with heavy metals in rats. Polish Journal of Environmental Studies. 2008;**17**(6):911-915

[33] Bystrická J, Vollmannová A, Musilová J. Ťažké kovy v systéme kontaminantov v chemickej toxikológii. Acta Facultatis Universitatis. Tym Avensis, Ser D. 2008;**2**(12):253-255

[34] Bencko V, Cikrt M, Lener J. Toxické kovy v životním a pracovním prostředí člověka. Praha: Grada Publishing; 1995. 282 p. ISBN 80-7169-150-X

[35] Kenedy S. Epidemiology: Why Can't we test our to absolute food safety? Science. 2008;**322**:1641-1643. DOI: 10.1126/science.1163867

[36] Svobodová Z, Máchová J, Vykusová B, Piačka V. Kovy v ekosystéme povrchových vod. Vodňany, Czech Republic: University of South Bohemia České Budějovice, Research Institute of Fish Culture and Hydrobiology; 1996. pp. 6-8. ISSN 0007-389X

[37] Cigánková V, Almášiová V, Holovská K. Morphological changes in Japanese quail duodenal epithelium after chronic cadmium exposure. Polish Journal of Environmental Studies. 2010;**19**(2):275-282

[38] Massanyi P, Lukáč N, Uhrín V, Toman R, Pivko J, Rafay J, et al. Female reproduktive toxicology of cadmium. Acta Biologica Hungarica. 2007;**58**:287-299

[39] ATSDR (Agency for Toxic Substances and Disease Registry). Toxicological Profile for Cadmium. U.S. Department of Health and Human Services; 2008. pp. 1-512. ISBN 978-92-9213-152

[40] Li Q, Cal S, Mo C, Chu B, Peng L, Yang F. Toxic effects of heavy metals and their accumulation in vegetables grown in a saline soil. Ecotoxicology and Environmental Safety. 2010;**73**:84-88

[41] Castellanos P, Reglero MM, Taggart MA, Mateo R. Changes in fatty acid profiles in testis and spermatoza of red deer exposed to metal pollution. Reproductive Toxicology. 2010;**29**:346-352

[42] Wirth JJ, Mijal RS. Adverse effects of low level heavy metal exposure on male reproductive function. Systems Biology in Reproductive Medicine. 2010;**56**:147-167

[43] Henson MC, Chedrese PJ. Endocrine Discruption by cadmium a common toxicants with paradoxical effects on reproduction. Experimental Biology and Medicine. 2004;**20**:181-185

[44] Lukáč N, Massányi P, Capcarová M, et al. Vplyv toxických kovov na imunitný systém. Potravinárstvo. 2009;**3**(3):35-38

[45] Bloom MS, Parsons PJ, Steuerwald AJ. Toxic trace metals and human oocytes during in vitro fertilization (IVF). Reproductive Toxicology. 2010:298-305

[46] Slivkova J, Massanyi P, Pizzi F, Trandzik J, Roychoudry S, Lukač N, et al. In vitro toxicity of mercuric chloride on rabbit spermatoza motility and cell membrane integrity. Journal Environtal Science Health A. 2010;**45**:767-774

[47] Babčan, J, Khun M, Sevc J. Toxicita ťažkých kovov - životné prostredie. Životné prostredie, revue pre teóriu a tvorbu ŽP. SAV Bratislava. vol. 5. 1999. pp. 1-5. ISBN 80-228-0869-5

[48] Bencko V et al. Hygiena. Praha; ČR: Nakladatelství Karolinum Praha; 2002. 205 p. ISBN 80-7184-551-5

[49] Bencko V, Cikrt M, Lener J. Toxické kovy v pracovním a životním prostředí

člověka. Praha: Avicenum, zdravotnické nakladatelství; 1985. p. 264. ISBN 80-7169-150-x

[50] Singh VK, Mishra KP, Rani R, Yaday VS, Awasthi SK, Garg SK. Immunomodulation by lead. Immunologic Research. 2003;**28**:151-166

[51] Zachar D. Výživa človeka I. Zvolen: TU, 2008. 328p. ISBN 80-85617-56-0

[52] CDC (Centers for Disease Control and Prevention). Fourth National Report on Human Exposure to Environmental Chemicals2009. pp. 176-242. ISBN 978-0-520-07107-0

[53] Jesenská M, Hiščáková M, Novotný J, Link R, Kováč G. Koncentrácia olova v krvnom sere mlieku a moči dojníc. In: Rizikové factory potravového reťazca III. Nitra, SP. 2003. pp. 51-52. ISBN 80-8069-282-3

[54] Adriano DC. Trace Elements in Terrestial Environments. 2nd ed. Springer; 2001. pp. 263-677. ISBN 0-387-98678-2

[55] Sinclair R, Boone SA, Greenberg D, Keim P, Gerba CHP. Persistence of category a slelect agents in the environment. Applied and Environmental Microbiology. 2008;**74**:555-663

[56] Ganga M. Hettiarachchi: Bioavailability, toxicity, and risk relationships in ecosystems. Environmental Quality. 2006;**5**:951-952

[57] Bíreš J, Húska M, Jenčík F. Chemické riziká potravinového reťazca v členských štátoch EÚ. In: Zb. XVII. vedecké sympózium s medzinárodnou účasťou, Hrádok. 2008. ISBN 987 80 970034 0 01. pp. 16-18

[58] Cimboláková I, Nováková J. Ťažké kovy - významná zložka potravového reťazca. Potravinárstvo. 2009;**3**(3): 14-16

[59] Cimboláková I, Nováková J, Lovásová E. Kadmium ako kontaminant vo vybraných potravinách. In: Bezpečnosť a kvalita surovín a potravín : V. vedecká konferencia s medzinárodnou účasťou. Nitra: Slovenská poľnohospodárska univerzita; 2010. ISBN 9788055203270. pp. 31-32

[60] Kimáková T, Kuzmova L, Bencko V, Nevolná Z. Fish and fish products as risk factors of mercury exposure. Annals of Agricultural and Environmental Medicine (AAEM). 2018;**25**(3): 488-493

[61] Tatiana K. Expozícia ortuťou z konzumácie rýb a rybích produktov. Lekársky obzor: odborný časopis Slovenskej zdravotníckej univerzity v Bratislave. 2018;**67**(3):110-114

[62] Sharpley A. Soil and water contamination: From molecular to catchment scale. Journal of Environmental Quality. 2007;**36**:607-608

[63] Frankovská J, Slaninka I. Environmentálne záťaže - stav riešenia v Európe a na Slovensku. Enviromagazín. 2009;**2**:4-7

[64] Ništiar F, Beňačka R, Rácz O. Základy molekulovej medicíny III. Košice: UPJŠ; 2005. pp. 1-69 80-7097-591-1

[65] Alloway BJ. Soil processes and the behaviour of metals. In: Alloway BJ, editor. Heavy Metals in Soil. London: Blackie Academic & Professional; 1995. 368 p. ISBN 0-751-401-986

[66] Baird C. Environmental Chemistry. New York: W.H. Freeman and Copany; 2004, . 652 p 9780716748779

[67] Sahmoun AE, Case LD, Jackson SA, Schwarz GG. Cadmium and prostate cancer: Acritical epidemiological analysis. Cancer Investigation. 2005;**23**:256-263

[68] Al-Najar H, Schulz R, Breuer J, Roemheld V. Effect of cropping systems on the mobilityand uptake of Cd and Zn. Environmental Chemistry Letters. 2005;**3**:13-17

[69] Kabata-Pendias A, Pendias H. Trace Elements in Soils and Plants. 3th ed. CRC Press; 2000. pp. 143-154. ISBN 978-1-4200-3990-0

[70] Šalgovičová D. Hodnotenie expozície kadmiom v podmienkach Slovenskej republiky: výskumná správa; 2009, pp. 1-31

[71] Richter R. Živinný režim rúd - ťežké kovy v púde. MZLU Brno: Ústav agrochemie a výživy rostlín; 2004. pp. 156-165

[72] EFSA (European Food Safety Authority). Cadmium in food. The EFSA Journal. 2009;**980**:1-139

[73] ATSDR (Agency for Toxic Substances and Disease Registry). Toxicological Profile for Mercury. U.S. Department of Health and Human Services; 1999. pp. 1-676. ISBN 1-888-422-8737

[74] Hayes W. Principles and Methods of Toxicology. Vol. 33. CRC Press; 2007. pp. 858-861. ISBN 9780849337789

[75] WHO. Air Quality Guidelines for Europe, 2000

[76] Křištofová D. Kovy a životní prostředí. Environmentálně nebezpečné složky elektroodpadu. 1st ed. Ostrava: VŠB-TU Ostrava; 2005. p. 66. ISBN 80-248-0740-8

[77] Issaro N, Abi-Ghanen C, Bermond A. Fractionation studies ofmercury in soils and sediments: A review of the chemical reagents used for mercury extraction. Analytica Chimica Acta. 2009;**631**(1):1-12

[78] Urban P. Aktuální problémy neurotoxicity rtuti. Neurológia pre Prax. 2006;**5**:251-253

[79] UNEP IOMC. United Ntions Environment Programme-Chemicals: Global Mercury Assessment. Inter-Organization Programme for the Sound Management of Chemicals. Ženeva; 2002. 258 p

[80] WHO. Environmental Health Criteria 86: Mercury – Environmental Aspects. Geneva; Published under the joint sponsorship of the United Nations Environment Programme, the International Labour Organisation, and the World Health Organization. ISBN 92-415-4286-1. 1989; 115 p

[81] Ďurža O, Khun M. Environmentálna geochémia niektorých ťažkých kovov. UK: Bratislava; 2002. 116 p. ISBN 80 223 1657 1

[82] Velíšek J. Chemie potravin 2.1. OSSIS: Pelhřimov; 1999. 328 p. ISBN 80-902391-4-5

[83] Kimáková T, Bernasovská K. Zaťaženie životného prostredia ortuťou na priemyselne exponovanom území Slovenska. Slovenský veterinársky časopis. 2005;**30**(6):369-370

[84] Mari M, Domingo JL. Toxic emission from crematories: A review. Environment International. 2010;**36**(1):131-137

[85] Tichý M. Toxikoloógie pro chemiky. Toxikoógie obecná, speciální, analytická a legislatíva. Praha: Karolinum; 2003, 2003. 119 p. ISBN 80-246-0566-X

[86] Kimáková T, Bernasovská K. Sledovanie koncentrácie ortuti vo vybraných potravinách. In: Využitie chemických metód pri ochrane a podpore zdravia obyvateľstva. Košice: UPJŠ; 2008. pp. 38-43. ISBN 9788070977279

[87] Gerhardsson L, Skerfving S. Concepts on biological markers and biomonitoring for metal toxicity. In:

Chang LW, Magos L, Suzuki T, editors. Toxicology of Metals. USA: CRC Press. Inc; 1996. pp. 81-107

[88] Pískač A, Kačmár P, Kol A. Veterinární toxikológie. Živočíšna výroba: Státní zemědelské nakladatelství v Praze ve spolupráci s nakladatelstvím Príroda v Brateslavě ve sbírce; 1985. p. 256. ISBN 80-7148-022-3

[89] Guzzi G, La Porta CA. Molecular mechanisms triggered by mercury. Toxicology. 2008;**244**(1):1-12

[90] Aschner M, Onishchenko N, Ceccatelli S. Toxicology of alkyl-mercury compuounds. In: Metal Ions Life Sciences. Vol. 7. 2010. pp. 403-434. ISBN 978-1-84755-177-1

[91] Ariza ME, Bijur GN, Williams MV. Lead and mercury mutagenesis: Role of H_2O_2, superoxide dismutase, and xanthine oxidase. Environmental and Molecular Mutagenesis. 1998;**31**:352-361

[92] Myers GJ, Davidson PW, Cox C, Shamlaye C, Cernichiari E, Clarkson TW. Twenty-seven years studying the human neurotoxicity of methylmercury exposure. Environmental Research. 2000;**83**(3):275-285

[93] Clarkson TW. The three modern faces of mercury. Environmental Health Perspectives. 2002;**110**:11-23

[94] Schober SE, Sinks TH, Jones RL, Bolger PM, Mcdowell M, Osterloh J. Blood mercury levels in US children and women of childbearing age, 1999-2000. JAMA. 2003;**289**(13):1667-1674

[95] AAP & USPHS. Joint statement of the American Academy of Pediatrics and the United States Public Health Service. Pediatrics. 1999;**104**:568-569

[96] USPHS - US Public Health Service, 1999. ISBN 05-20253-76-0.

[97] Ball LK, Ball R, Pratt RD. An assessment of thimerosal use in childhood vaccines. Pediatrics. 2001;**107**(5):1147-1154

[98] Magos L. Review on the toxicity of ethylmercury, including its presence as a preservative in biological and pharmaceutical products. Journal of Applied Toxicology. 2001;**21**(1):1-5

[99] Tuček M. Současná zdravotní rizika expozice rtuti a jejim sloučeninám. České pracovní lékařství. 2006;**7**(1):26-34

[100] IARC (International Agency for Research on Cancer). Cadmium and cadmium compounds. Berylium, cadmium, mercury, and exposures in the glass manufacturing industry. In: IARC Monographs on the Evalution of Carcnogenetic Risks to Humans. Vol. 58. 1993, 1993. pp. 119-237

Chapter 4

Sanitation and the Environment

Mária Vargová, Katarína Veszelits Laktičová, Rudolf Hromada, Iveta Cimboláková, Ivan Uher, Ingrid Papajová and Korim Peter

Abstract

The environment is severything that creates natural conditions for the existence of organisms, including humans, and is a prerequisite for its further development. Proper environmental hygiene can prevent the outbreak and spread of infectious diseases. The function of disinfectants is to kill and prevent the growth of microorganisms. Disinfectants are potentially noxious substances which are used in intensive animal production and disease control programmes. In fulfilling this role, disinfectants may also have an adverse impact on the environment. These products may harm beneficial microorganisms, plant and animal life, and even humans, when used without due caution. Proper selection of disinfectant which is based on the knowledge of the resistance of microorganisms to the effect of the disinfectant and the efficacy of the disinfectants as well as the potential negative impact on the environment minimizes the risk of microbiological contamination and improves quality of the environment.

Keywords: sanitation, microorganisms, environment, disinfection, hygiene, disinfectants

1. Introduction

One of the most significant environmental problems of the present, affecting all environmental components, is global environmental contamination, which is closely linked to the unprecedented boom in industrial and agricultural chemistry. The environment, both natural and artificial, is one of the factors that affect human health and well-being. The relationship between the environment and health, the so-called environmental health, should be understood as a complex of interactions between the genetic characteristics of a human being and the environment in which she lives. Exposure of men to environmental pollutants can trigger the onset of diseases, most often chronic [1]. Environmental contamination plays an important role in the transmission of several key health care-associated pathogens. Effective and thorough cleaning/disinfecting of the patient environment is essential. Although microbiologically contaminated surfaces can serve as reservoirs of potential pathogens, these surfaces generally are not directly associated with transmission of infections to either staff or patients. The transferral of microorganisms from environmental surfaces to patients is largely via hand contact with the surface. Although hand hygiene is important to minimize the impact of this transfer, cleaning and disinfecting environmental surfaces as appropriate is fundamental in reducing their potential contribution to the incidence of healthcare-associated infections.

The principles of cleaning and disinfecting environmental surfaces take into account the intended use of the surface or item in patient care [2]. Protecting human, animal and plant healthiness at every stage of the food production process is one of the top priorities for the public health and economy. Food safety is becoming increasingly of interest to consumers and producers, and microbiological purity of food raw materials, technological equipment, production areas and final products is inseparably linked to it. Therefore, a great emphasis is placed on the whole quality assurance complex, including production hygiene [3]. Foodborne diseases encompass a wide spectrum of illnesses and are a growing public health problem worldwide. They are the result of ingestion of foodstuffs contaminated with microorganisms or chemicals. The contamination of food may occur at any stage in the process from food production to consumption ("farm to fork") and can result from environmental contamination, including pollution of water, soil or air [4]. Environmental sanitation is the promotion of hygiene and the prevention of disease and other consequences of ill-health, relating to environmental factors. To allow for transmission of infectious agents they have to be present in the immediate human environment, exposure has to take place, and transmission has to occur by uptake of the agents through unsafe practices. To interrupt the transmission, environmental sanitation can act on reducing exposure to infectious agents by limiting contact to wastes or polluted media, and by changing hygiene and socio-cultural practices. Sanitation is the effective use of tools and actions that keep our environment healthy. Sanitation is a complex of measures directed to the inactivation, removal, or killing of the agents of infections in the external environment. Sanitation includes disinfection, insect control, rodent control, proper disposal of wastes (cadavers, excrements, wastewater) and hygiene of the environment [5].

2. Disinfection

Disinfection is defined as a process in which germs are destroyed by either chemical action or physical intervention, or a combination of both [6].

2.1 Stages of disinfection

Disinfection has several stages. The first stage is the **exploratory and preparatory work** to determine the extent and type of disinfected object. The necessary amount of tools, aids, appliances, employees and effective disinfectant must be provided [7]. Cleaning, second stage, is the necessary first step of any disinfection process. Cleaning removes organic matter, salts, and visible soils, all of which interfere with microbial inactivation. The physical action of scrubbing with detergents and surfactants and rinsing with water removes substantial numbers of microorganisms. If a surface is not cleaned first, the success of the disinfection process can be compromised. Removal of all visible blood and inorganic and organic matter can be as critical as the germicidal activity of the disinfecting agent. When a surface cannot be cleaned adequately, it should be protected with barriers. It has been estimated that cleaning alone may remove over 90% of bacteria from surfaces [8]. The third stage is the **actual disinfection**, its objective being to destroy the decisive number of microorganisms that remained on the objects and surfaces after mechanical cleaning. The fourth stage is **to check the effectiveness of disinfection**. The effectiveness of surface disinfection must be controlled. The inspection informs about the quality of the work done and about the effectiveness of the disinfectants used. In the case of identified insufficiencies, it is the basis for the implementation of corrective measures. The effectiveness of disinfection is checked by chemical and microbiological swabs. Chemical methods are divided into qualitative and quantitative. The methods are very costly and time consuming, thus they are rarely done. Methods are currently available to detect undesirable residues of disinfectants on surfaces as well as in products. Microbiological swabs can be used to verify that microorganisms have been killed on disinfected areas and objects [9]. The fifth stage is **ventilation and deactivation**. This stage is only performed after the disinfectant exposure time necessary for action has expired. Residues of disinfectants on surfaces and objects are removed through rinsing with water; in some cases, inactivating substances are used. A protocol shall be drawn up after each disinfection carried out [10].

2.2 Environmental factors influencing the effectiveness of disinfection

The effectiveness of disinfectants for microorganisms depends on many factors. On the one hand, these are the properties of the microorganisms themselves, on the other hand, the chemical and physical properties of the external environment. Knowing these factors should lead to a more adequate use of disinfection. The number and types of microorganisms present on environmental surfaces are influenced by the following factors:

a. number of people in the environment

b. amount of activity

c. amount of moisture

d. presence of material capable of supporting microbial growth

e. rate at which organisms suspended in the air are removed

f. type of surface and orientation (e.g. horizontal or vertical) [10].

Factors that affect disinfection efficiency include:

- the concentration of the disinfectant
- the time during which the microorganism is in contact with the disinfectant
- pH
- temperature
- the presence of organic contaminants, e.g., blood, serum or other body fluids
- the microorganism itself or the respective agent, their type (prions, viruses, gram-negative, gram-positive bacteria, microscopic fungi, protozoa, spores) as well as their number and location [11].

The most important factor is the concentration of the disinfectant from which the effectiveness of the disinfection depends. The mechanism of action depends on the chemical composition of the disinfectant and the way it is used. In the case of unstable disinfectants (chlorinated lime, formalin, Persteril), the concentration of active substance must be utaken into account when preparing the working solution. Inadequate (too low) concentration of the disinfectant used does not achieve a cidal effect, but only bacteriostatic, virostatic, and similar ones. Too high concentrations damage the disinfected objects and also lead to increased disinfection costs [9]. The pH values of the environment in which the disinfectant reacts with the microorganism is also an important factor affecting the final result. For example, glutaraldehyde and quaternary ammonium salts as well as chlorhexidine have higher efficacy at alkaline pH. On the other hand, phenolic preparations as well as chlorine are more effective at acidic pH. The temperature, in particular its increase, also partialy affects the end result of the disinfectant reaction with the microorganism [11]. At a low temperature of disinfectant solutions, dissociation of some disinfectants slows down, thereby reducing their diffusion into the bacterial cell. Some disinfectants (lyes) work better if they are heated to 70–80°C (in addition to chemical, they have physical effects too). Chloramine solutions are most effective at the temperature of 50–60°C [9]. The environmental pollutants of organic origin in which chemical disinfection is to be applied significantly reduce the activity of the disinfectant [11]. The presence of organic substances in the environment reduces the effect of all disinfectants; therefore, as previously mentioned before the disinfection of the object, it is necessary to clean the environment [9]. Microorganisms differ in their resistance to disinfectants. Different types of microoganisms vary in there responses to antiseptics, disinfectants, and sterilants (**Figure 1**). This is hardly surprising, in view of there different cellular structures, compositions, and physiologies. Traditionally, microbial susceptibilities to biocides have been classified based on these differences. Bacterial spores are generally considered the organisms most resistant to antiseptics, disinfectants, and strilants, although prions have shown market resistance to many physical and chemical processes. It is important to note that this classification is considered only a general guide to antimicrobial activity and can vary depending on the biocide, formulation, or process under consideration [11].

	Microorganism	Examples
More Resistant	Prions	Scrapie, Creutzfeldt-Jakob disease, chronic wasting disease
	Bacterial spores	*Bacillus, Geobacillus, Clostridium*
	Protozoal oocysts	*Cryptosporidium*
	Helminth eggs	*Ascaris, Enterobius*
	Mycobacteria	*Mycobacterium tuberculosis, M. terrae, M. chelonae*
	Small, nonenveloped viruses	Poliovirus, parvoviruses, papillomaviruses
	Protozoal cysts	*Giardia, Acanthamoeba*
	Fungal spores	*Aspergillus, Penicillium*
	Gram-negative bacteria	*Pseudomonas, Providencia, Escherichia*
	Vegetative fungi and algae	*Aspergillus, Trichophyton, Candida, Chlamydomonas*
	Vegetative helminths and protozoa	*Ascaris, Cryptosporidium, Giardia*
	Large, nonenveloped viruses	Adenoviruses, rotaviruses
	Gram-positive bacteria	*Staphylococcus, Streptococcus, Enterococcus*
Less Resistant	Enveloped viruses	Human immunodeficiency virus, hepatitis B virus, herpes simplex virus

Figure 1.
Decreasing order of resistance of microorganisms to disinfection and sterilization and the level of disinfection or sterilization. source: McDonnell, 2007.

2.3 Biofilm

Biofilms are composed of immobilized bacteria deposited in an organic polymeric mass of bacterial origin. Biofilm cells are irreversibly connected to each other and with the surface via extracellular polymeric substances (EPS), which account for up to 85% of the total biofilm mass. EPS include a number of proteins, glycoproteins, glycolipids, and in some cases a surprising amount of extracellular DNA [12]. Extracellular polymers are produced by bacteria that allow bacteria to adhere to the surface. The polymeric products constitute the base matrix. Biofilm further contains substances that belong to the "*quorum sensing*" (QS) system that is involved in intercellular bacterial communication.

Biofilm formation is a dynamic process that includes the following steps:

- surface attachment

- the formation of a monolayer

- differentiation of microcolonies

- differentiation of macrocolonies and ultimately a mature form of biofilm being created [13]. Various nutrients in the wet environment absorbed on the surfaces create an acclimation coating with different physico-chemical properties. The physico-chemical properties of the surface determine how the bacteria attach. The structure of the biofilm is not homogeneous; it contains a set of numerous channels and cavities that serve to circulate water, supply nutrients and oxygen. They are intricate, mutually communicating channels of various shapes that supply substances and gases to biofilm-living bacteria. Bacteria in the biofilm form clusters of cells, which are known as microcolonies. Biofilm architecture is diverse, constantly changing in space and time due to external and internal processes. It is known that EPS production and hence the related biofilm thickness depend on the availability of nutrients and whether the biofilm is composed of one or more bacterial species. In a natural environment, the community of several species is more common. Biofilm formation is a cause of problems in many areas, e.g. in medicine, in water supply systems, in the food production industry [12]. Biofilm for microorganisms in a given environment creates both a nutritional layer that allows for their reproduction and a protective layer that limits the devitalizing effects of the disinfectants used. Thus, prevention is effective cleaning and application of combined compositions, e.g., oxidizing agents, surfactants and regular surface monitoring. The intervals needed; the intensity of cleaning and decontamination depend on the degree of contamination that occurs on different surfaces [14].

2.3.1 Methods of biofilm removal

The removal of impurities from surfaces must be of a high standard to ensure technological and hygienic requirements. In general, we distinguish three types of biofilm removal:

- mechanical

- chemical

- biological [15].

Physical methods (otherwise called mechanical methods) are based on the action of a magnetic field that is highly intense. Ultrasonic devices (high-frequency electric field devices) or their connection with organic acids are used. Chemical methods consist of using detergents and disinfectants the acting of which is necessary to effectively remove biofilms. Significant is the use of ozone and a variety of chlorine-based preparations, iodine compounds, peroxyacetic acid, and quaternary ammonium compounds [13]. Biological methods degrade biofilms using enzymes produced by bacteria, but their use is limited because of their cost and affordability. In order to achieve the desired effect, it is appropriate to use a combination of methods with a synergistic effect.

2.4 Chemical disinfection

Disinfectants are classified by their chemical nature and each class has its unique characteristics, hazards, toxicities and efficacy against various microorganisms. Environmental conditions, such as the presence of organic matter, pH or water hardness can also impact the action of the disinfectant [10].

Different disinfectants have different mechanisms of action, all disinfectants act by harming microorganisms in some manner. Mechanisms of harm include:

1. Protein denaturation

2. Membrane disruption

3. Nucleic acid damage

4. Inhibition of metabolism [16].

The ideal disinfectant must have a wide range of action, rapid, time-saving use, and water solubility. The disinfectant should also be stable, ecological, non-toxic, non-corrosive, economical and safe to use. However, such a disinfectant does not exist in real practice and it is therefore important to choose a suitable combination of disinfectants. Rotation of disinfectants is good practice. The mechanism of action of disinfectants on microorganisms can generally be divided into four categories:

- denaturation of proteins

- membrane damage

- damage of nucleic acids

- inhibition of metabolic activity.

Disinfectants are placed into three categories depending on microbicidal activity:

- High-level disinfectants

- Intermediate-level disinfectants

- Low-level disinfectants [17].

High-level disinfectants (HLD) are active against vegetative bacteria, viruses (including the nonenveloped ones), fungi, and mycobacteria. They may also have some activity against bacterial spores with extended contact times. Aldehydes (glutaraldehyde and ortho-phthalaldehyde) and oxidisers (e.g., hydrogen peroxide and peracetic acid) are HLDs. The aldehydes are non-corrosive and safe for use on most devices. However, they can fix organic materials; therefore, it is particularly important to remove any embedded microbes prior to disinfection. Unless properly formulated and carefully used, oxidisers can be corrosive. However, they can be faster-acting, non-fixative, and safer for the environment than aldehydes. HLDs typically require 10–45 min of contact time for disinfection, depending on the temperature. After disinfection, items require thorough rinsing with sterile or filtered water to remove any chemical residues; they must then be dried with an alcohol rinse or by blowing clean and filtered air through the device's channels prior to safe storage. A disinfectant (e.g., ethanol) is active against vegetative bacteria, mycobacteria, fungi, and most viruses. It may fail to kill spores, even after prolonged exposure. Low-level disinfectants (e.g., quaternary ammonium compounds) are active against vegetative bacteria (except mycobacteria), some fungi, and only enveloped viruses. In many cases, washing with unmedicated soap and water would be sufficient in place of such disinfectants [18]. There are three levels of disinfection: high, intermediate, and low. High-level disinfectants, such as glutaraldehyde, are used as chemical sterilants and should never be used on environmental surfaces. Intermediate-level disinfectants are registered with the Environmental Protection Agency (EPA) and have a tuberculocidal claim, and low-level disinfectants are EPA-registered without a tuberculocidal claim (i.e., hepatitis B virus and HIV label claims). The process of high-level disinfection, an appropriate standard of treatment for heat-sensitive, semicritical medical instruments (e.g., flexible, fiberoptic endoscopes), inactivates all vegetative bacteria, mycobacteria, viruses, fungi, and some bacterial spores. High-level disinfection is accomplished with powerful, sporicidal chemicals (e.g., glutaraldehyde, peracetic acid, and hydrogen peroxide) that are not appropriate for use on housekeeping surfaces. These liquid chemi cal sterilants/high-level disinfectants are highly toxic. Use of these chemicals for applications other than those indicated in their label instructions (i.e., as immersion chemicals for treating heat-sensitive medical instruments) is not appropriate [17]. Intermediate-level disinfection does not necessarily kill bacterial spores, but it does inactivate *Mycobacterium tuberculosis* var. bovis, which is substantially more resistant to chemical germicides than ordinary vegetative bacteria, fungi, and medium to small viruses (with or without lipid envelopes). Chemical germicides with sufficient potency to achieve intermediate-level disinfection include chlorine-containing compounds (e.g., sodium hypochlorite), alcohols, some phenolics, and some iodophors [18]. Low-level disinfection inactivates vegetative bacteria, fungi, enveloped viruses, e.g., human immunodeficiency virus (HIV) and influenza viruses, and some non-enveloped viruses (e.g., adenoviruses). Low-level disinfectants include quaternary ammonium compounds, some phenolics, and some iodophors [2]. The health and safety of humans and animals should always be a primary consideration when selecting a disinfectant. Most disinfectants have some level of hazard associated with their use. Some pose a serious threat to human and animal health (i.e., aldehydes, phenols, sodium hydroxide). Some cannot be used when animals are present or must be thoroughly rinsed away with potable water prior to restocking. Personnel training, personal protective measures and safety precautions should always be taken. Environmental factors, such as runoff into creeks or ponds, must also be considered when selecting a disinfectant. Many agents are known ecological hazards for plants and aquatic life (i.e., sodium carbonate, hypochlorites, phenolic compounds), therefore drainage, runoff, and biodegradability of disinfectants should be considered [19].

2.4.1 Chemical disinfectants

Chemical disinfectants are chemical agents applied to non-living objects in order to destroy bacteria, viruses, fungi, mold or mildews living on the objects. By definition, disinfectant formulas must be registered with the Environmental Protection Agency (EPA). The "active ingredient" in each disinfectant formula is what kills pathogens, usually by disrupting or damaging their cells [20].

2.4.1.1 Alkalis

Alkalis (or bases) are defined as substances capable of forming hydroxide (OH^-) ions when dissolved in water and are measured at pH > 7. Hydroxides are strong bases with a pH above 12 and are very reliable disinfectants. Alkalis have good microbicidal properties; inhibit the growth of microorganisms by restricting various metabolic processes. In general, pH values of ≥9 are restrictive for the growth of most vegetative microorganisms, including bacteria and fungi. Low concentrations are generally inhibitory, while higher concentrations are bactericidal and fungicidal. Typical virucidal concentrations are 1–2% NaOH [21]. The mechanism of action of the hydroxide is based on changing the pH of the environment. The reaction of alkali with the various types of lipids (including phospolipids) in these membranes can be compared to their reactions with fatty acids in lipids and oils to cause salt (soap) formation. Membrane disruption leads to cell wall destabilization and loss of membrane structure and function, including disruption of the proton motive force and leakage of cytoplasmatic materials. Alkali also causes breakage of peptide bonds and the breakdown of proteins, which is presumed to be the major mechanism of action against prions [22]. Alkalis are very corrosive agents and damage to various surfaces, depending on the concentration of alkali used and the formulation pH. Personal protection precautions should be observed while working with alkalis [21]. Some limited disinfection methods use high concentrations of strong alkalis, such as NaOH (commonly known as caustic soda or soda lye) and KOH (also known as lye), while lower concentrations of these and weaker alkalis, such as sodium bicarbonate (baking soda) and sodium matasilicate, are used in various cleaning applications [23].

Potassium hydroxide (KOH) is used to produce greasy antiseptic soaps [24].

Sodium hydroxide (NaOH) is a strong surface disinfectant which finds a use in many farm situations [21]. The disinfecting effect of the lye depends on the concentration of hydroxyl ions. Sodium hydroxide has a moderately wide range of action. At concentrations of 3–5%, it has bactericidal effects, especially on gram-negative rods. The effect on cocci is not sufficient. Already at a 2% concentration it has a good virucidal effect on most viruses. Sodium hydroxide does not act well on mycobacterial rods and fungi [24]. A high concentration of this substance can kill all microorganisms including bacterial spores. Such concentrations will produce a pH of 13 or higher [21]. NaOH is stored in well-closed containers because it reacts with CO_2 in the air and thus loses efficiency, so freshly prepared hydroxide solutions should be used. It is well soluble in hot water (e.g., in water 18°C warm it dissolves to 51%, but in water heated to 70–80°C up to 75%), producing heat, as a side effect. It dissociates in water into negatively charged hydroxyl ions and positively charged sodium ions. Sodium hydroxide is highly corrosive and irritating to the skin, eyes and mucous membrane s of animals and humans; contact could result in severe burns. Most problems occur after careless use of this disinfectant [21]. Sodium hydroxide is a corrosive with a good deep effect [24]. Extreme caution is required when handling NaOH. Great care must be taken regarding the environmental impact of this product, especially when dealing with water run-off, as sodium hydroxide may severely affect the pH of surface water and plant life. It is recommended that this disinfectant be used only when there is absolute certainty that the environment will not be negatively affected. However, NaOH has the advantage of being relatively cheap and lends itself to being handled in bulk [21].

Calcium hydroxide Ca(OH)2 is prepared from burnt lime by slaking with water. A 20% suspension (lime milk) is prepared from freshly slaked lime. Slaked lime absorbs air carbon dioxide and turns into calcium carbonate, which is ineffective as disinfectant. The suspension prepared from freshly slaked lime has both viral and bactericidal effect [9].

2.4.1.2 Acids

Acids are defined as substances that dissociate in water to provide hydrogen ions (H^+), which are measured on the pH scale as <7 [25]. The effect of acids and their derivatives is based on the action of hydrogen ions, anions or whole molecules, surface activity, oxidative or dehydrating capabilities. Acidic disinfectants function by destroying the bonds of nucleic acids and precipitating proteins [21]. Acids also change the pH of the environment of cell, cause oxidaze a dehydratation as well as the destruction of fermentative metabolism of bacteria [26]. The effectiveness of the acids is reduced by the presence of organic contamination. Disadvantages of organic acids are their ability to interact with organic substances, thereby reducing their disinfectant activity, etching and corrosiveness [27]. The use of inorganic acids is considerably limited due to their corrosive and irritant effects. Of inorganic acids, hydrochloric acid, nitric acid and phosphoric acid are used in the disinfection practice [9].

Hydrochloric acid (HCl) is used in the form of *Schattenfroh solution*. The solution contains 2.5% hydrochloric acid and 15% cooking salt. It is used to disinfect anthrax – contaminated skin [21].

Nitric acid (HNO3) has a good sporocidal effect. It is used at a 2% concentration for bristle disinfection at 2 h exposure and a solution temperature of 40°C. After disinfection is complete, the bristles are neutralized with a 2% sodium hydroxide solution. A concentration of 0.3–0.5% at a solution temperature of 50°C is recommended today mainly for cleaning and disinfection of milking equipment in organic farming [28].

Phosphoric acid (H3PO4) is used to disinfect soil and manure at a concentration of 1.5–3%. Of the organic acids, peracetic acid and lactic acid are used in disinfection practice.

Peracetic acid (CH3COOH) is the most potent of the above-mentioned substances, acting in a bactericidal, sporocidal, viricidal and fungicidal way. Peracetic acid is part of Persteril, a composition which contains 32–36% peracetic acid, 7–10% hydrogen peroxide, 1% sulfuric acid. Persteril is an unstable preparation and is prepared for the active substance content [29].

Peracetic acid is oxidizing agents, denatures proteins, disrupts cell wall permeability, and oxidizes sulfhydral and sulfur bonds in proteins, enzymes, and other metabolites [27]. Its advantage is that it works at low concentrations. At a concentration of 0.4%, it acts on the surfaces after a 30 min exposure. Persteril as a 0.1% solution is used to treat growing mold directly on the meat. For hand disinfection it is used as a 1–0.2% solution. It leaves no residue, rapidly decomposes into acetic acid and water. Peracetic acid is used to disinfect the environment, surfaces and medical devices. In the form of an aerosol or spray, Pedox-PAA50, which contains 10–40% peracetic acid, is the most commonly applied formulation. For aerosol disinfection, it is used in the concentration of 5–7 ml m^{-3}. The disadvantages of using peracetic acid include corrosion to metals. Even this disadvantage can be avoided by the addition of sodium pyrophosphate in the ratio 1:2 to peracetic acid. It has to be stored at a temperature below 20°C. It is best stored in a refrigerator at 4°C [29].

Lactic acid is mainly used to disinfect air in the presence of animals. It is used in the form of an aerosol, in an amount of 5 ml m^{-3} [30].

2.4.1.3 Halogens

Halogen-containing disinfectants include chlorine, iodine, bromine and fluorine preparations, which are the most reactive and the most toxic of the halogen compounds. Halogen-containing compounds which are toxic to the cell are created by the action of oxygen in the initial phase. The optimum pH for the disinfection effect is 5–8 and the presence of organic substances significantly reduces it. For practical disinfection, iodine, chlorine and its compounds are important [31].

2.4.1.4 Iodine and iodonal

The position and importance of iodine among the disinfectants lies in its intense and, above all, rapid action on all microorganisms at quite low toxicity. Iodine is a crystalline substance that sublimes at normal temperature and pressure. However, aqueous or alcoholic iodine solutions carry many undesirable effects and their wider use in disinfection was hindered by their significant negative properties such as low solubility in water, corrosion, staining of disinfected objects, toxicity, and the like [9]. Iodine-based disinfectants are called iodophores. Iodophores are relatively non-toxic. In iodophores, iodine is bound to polyvinylpyrrolidones (surface-active organic polymers), which have a significant effect on increasing the disinfection efficiency of these formulations.

Iodine compounds are broad spectrum and considered effective for a variety of bacteria, mycobacteria, fungi and viruses [23]. The negative properties of iodophores are considerably limited, have corrosive effects on iron, less affect copper and its compounds. They have a weak corrosive effect on zinc, aluminum and tin. They do not rust stainless steel. At long-term use, they leave stains and color PVC (polyvinyl chloride) and polyethylene. Iodophores are water-soluble, stable, non-allergenic, fast-acting, low-toxicity, and non-irritating to injured skin. When using iodophores, the basic requirement, namely a thorough mechanical cleansing, must be fulfilled. The temperature of the solutions should not exceed 35°C [32]. They are used in healthcare, veterinary care, food production industry, agriculture and municipal hygiene. Iodine preparations can be used both to disinfect surfaces and to disinfect skin as antiseptics.

Jodonal A contains 1.75% active iodine, 12.5% phosphoric acid and a stabilizer. It has viracidal, sporocidal and bactericidal effects, also against acid-resistant mycobacteria. It is used in the food production industry.

Jodonal B contains 1.65% active iodine, 3.6% phosphoric acid and a stabilizer. Jodonal B is used in health care and municipal hygiene.

Jodonal M contains 1.6% iodine, followed by citric acid and glycerin, which has a protective effect on mucous membranes. Jodonal M is used in the prevention of mastitis in cows, is designed for disinfection of teats after milking at 20% concentration. It is used for udder treatment in 2–4% concentration [9].

2.4.1.5 Chlorine and its compounds

Chlorine preparations are widely used. Chlorine is responsible for the major mechanism of action and thus the inactivation of enzymes and ribosome proteins, due to the formation of a strong oxidizing agent – HClO (hypochlorous acid), which is the result of the reaction of chlorine with water. The bacterial cell undergoes changes in the cytoplasmic membrane, the oxidation of thiol groups of enzymes and chlorination of nucleotides occurs, resulting in the blockade of DNA synthesis [33]. An important element is chlorine, occurring in the form of poisonous yellow-brown gas. Chlorination is the most widely used method for disinfecting water supplies. The disinfecting ability of chlorine in water depends on the degree of its dissociation. In an acidic environment, their disinfection effect increases. Chlorine preparations contain salts of hypochlorous acid (HClO). Their decomposition in aqueous environment produces hydrochloric acid (HCl) and oxygen in the phase of "birth," which oxidizes organic substances. The chemical activity of the chlorine preparations is associated with the chlorine found together with the oxygen in the hypochlorite group -ClO. The amount of oxygen released by the decomposition of this group corresponds to the content of reactive chlorine in a preparation called as active chlorine. Thus, active chlorine is an indicator of disinfectant properties in chlorine preparations. The active chlorine content in the chlorine preparations is expressed as a percentage. Chlorine preparations belong to the group of oxidizing agents with very good disinfection effect [34, 35]. Chlorine compounds are inactivated by organic soil, so a cleaning step is often required for heavily soiled surfaces. They are also prone to degradation from exposure to heat, UV light, and transition metals, such as copper, nickel, cobalt, and iron [36]. Activated solutions are recommended for disinfection especially for mycobacteria and spore-forming bacteria. In the food producing industry, it is not recommended to disinfect the surfaces with which the raw materials or food come into direct contact with chlorine preparations. The effect of all chlorine derivatives is accelerated by the addition of ammonia and ammonium salts, which is the essence of so-called activation of chlorine preparations. However, this activation is short-lived so that the activated solutions must be used immediately, especially against the highly resistant microbes. Ammonium salts, in the ratio 1:1 and ammonia, in the ratio 1:8 to 16 [9] are added to the solutions of known concentration. The most commonly used chlorine preparations include chloramines, chlorinated lime, dikonit, sodium hypochlorite.

Chloramines are organic compounds containing 25–30% active chlorine. Chloramines are stable powder substances, well soluble, with corrosive and whitening effects. They have bactericidal, fungicidal and virucidal activity. At alkaline pH, their effect decreases rapidly. In disinfection practice, Chloramine T is the most significant. In aqueous solution it hydrolyses more slowly than chlorinated lime, explaining its more gentle action on fabrics, metals, wood and other disinfected materials. Chloramine T is a relatively stable preparation. Losses of active chlorine when stored correctly are only 0.1% per year. Chloramine T solutions heated up to 50–60°C are more effective than non-heated solutions. Chloramine T has a bactericidal effect, while higher concentrations (10%) are required for mycobactericidal action in practical disinfection. Preventive disinfection uses a 2–3% solution, 4–10% for focal disinfection [9].

Fresh chlorinated lime contains 33–36% of active chlorine. It dissolves only partially in water. It is unstable in air and must be stored in impermeable, well sealed containers, dry and protected from light. The effectiveness of chlorinated lime is reduced by storage. It is used for wastewater disinfection, coarse disinfection and 2–3% for floor disinfection at 30 min. Exposure or till dry. Chlorinated lime has a good bactericidal effect, also against acid-resistant mycobacteria, further sporocidal effect, which can be enhanced by acidification with sulfuric acid, as well as a good virucidal activity. For practical disinfection, cold clarified solutions containing 1–2% of active chlorine are prepared. Chlorinated lime is used to disinfect farm buildings, cowsheds, paddocks, fences and cesspools [37].

Dikonit is a granular highly effective disinfectant preparation of chlorinated cyanuric acid containing at least 55% of active chlorine. It dissolves well in water. The solid surfaces are disinfected with 1–2% solution. Dikonit has the widest use in health care and community hygiene. In terms of its effect on microorganisms, it has bactericidal, fungicidal, virucidal, tuberculocidal effect.

Other representatives include **sodium hypochlorite**. Sodium hypochlorite is also called "liquid chlorine", which has bactericidal and virucidal properties.

2.4.1.6 Aldehydes

Aldehydes are highly effective, broad spectrum disinfectants, cause against bacteria, fungi, viruses, mycobacteria and spores [23]. The mechanism of action of aldehydes is based on protein denaturation and disrupting of nucleic acids [38]. The most commonly used agents are formaldehyde and gluteraldehyde. Aldehydes are non-corrosive to metals, rubber, plastic and cement [39]. These chemicals are highly irritating, toxic to humans or animals, therefore their use is limited [40].

Formaldehyde is an irritating gas dissolving in water into a nearly 40% solution called formalin. It has excellent microbicidal effects, reliably destroys bacteria, spores, fungi and viruses. It is used for surface disinfection at 2–3% concentration. It is also used as an aerosol. In special devices, formaldehyde mixed with water vapor at 60–80°C can be used to sterilize some instruments and delicate items. The disadvantage is its irritating odor almost to toxicity [10]. Formaldehyde has been classified by the International Agency for Cancer Research as a Group 1 Carcinogen, i.e. a proven human carcinogen. In view of the carcinogenic and teratogenic effect, formaldehyde used for a long time has been restricted in use, but is still used for sterilization in chemical autoclaves; however, it must be ensured that its vapors are sucked out of the environment so that the operator of the device is protected.

Glutaraldehyde is primarily used as a disinfectant for medical equipment (e.g., endoscopes), but can provide sterilization at prolonged contact times [38]. Glutaraldehyde has a broad spectrum of activity against bacteria and their spores, fungi, and viruses. Bacterial studies demonstrated a strong binding of glutaraldehyde to outer layers of organisms such as *E.coli* and *Staphylococcus aureus* [21]. A 2% concentration is used for highlevel disinfection. Its efficacy is highly dependant on pH and temperature, working best at a pH greater than 7 and high temperatures. It is considered more efficacious in the presence of organic matter, soaps and hard water than formaldehyde [38, 40].

2.4.1.7 Alcohol

The most feasible explanation for the antimicrobial action of alcohol is denaturation of proteins. Protein denaturation also is consistent with observations that alcohol destroys the dehydrogenases of *Escherichia coli*, and that ethyl alcohol increases the lag phase of *Enterobacter aerogenes* and that the lag phase effect could be reversed by adding certain amino acids. The bacteriostatic action was believed caused by inhibition of the production of metabolites essential for rapid cell division [21].

2.4.1.8 Surfactants

Surfactants from the Latin "*tensio*" are surface active substances that reduce the surface tension of liquids. According to the polar group, surfactants are divided into two basic groups, ionogenic and non-ionic. Ionogenic surfactants contain functional groups that dissociate in aqueous solution, thereby producing negative (anionic) or positive (cationic) charged ions. Their charge depends on the pH of the environment. Non-ionic surfactants are substances that do not dissociate in aqueous solution. Anionic surfactants include detergents and sulfonate detergents. Cationic surfactants have a bactericidal effect in addition to cleaning and wetting properties [41]. They act better in the alkaline environment, they are not corrosive and do not irritate the skin, also non-toxic, colorless, odorless and stable in the presence of organic material. Quaternary ammonium compounds are the most important class of surfactants that exhibit strong disinfectant effects. The best-known preparations are Ajatin and Septonex [9].

Ajatin is an effective disinfectant that acts on vegetative bacteria, the disadvantage of which is its low potency against spores and tuberculosis agents. It is used in 1% concentration for hand disinfection and in 5% concentration for skin disinfection. If we increase its concentration to 10%, it can only wash the hands for 3 min. The action of Ajatin consists in disrupting bacterial membranes and structures, inhibiting the metabolism of bacteria and causing denaturation of proteins and enzymes.

Septonex is a white powder, used as a 1% solution for hand, object and laundry disinfection [42].

2.5 Physical disinfection

Physical disinfection is based on the effect of physical quantities on the pathogenic microorganism. One of the variables is the exposure time, which precisely determines the time interval during which another physical quantity (temperature, wavelength, etc.) must act.

2.5.1 UV radiation

Ultraviolet germicidal radiation is an established means of disinfection and can be used to prevent the spread of certain infectious diseases. UV radiation is used to control airborne microorganisms and environmental surface decontamination [39]. The main sources of UV radiation are simple UV lights, including mercury vapor lamos, fluorescent lights, pulsed UV lamps, and "black – light" lamps [21]. Not all UV wavelenghts are effective against microorganisms (**Figure 2**). A main characteristic of UV light is that a specific range of its wavelengths, those between 200 and 300 nm, are categorized as germicidal, they are capable of inactivating bacteria, viruses and protozoa. This capability allows widespread adoption of UV light as a chemical-free, environmentally friendly and highly effective way to safeguard and disinfect water against harmful microorganisms [43]. The most effective

UV type	Common name	Wavelength range (nm)	Comments
UV-A	Long wave	315–400	Fluorescent light, black light
UV-B	Medium wave	280–315	Responsible for sunburn
UV-C	Short wave	200–280	Germicidal range

Figure 2.
Types of UV radiation. Source: McDonnell, 2007.

wavelenght has been found to be 265 nm [21]. Unlike chemical approaches to water disinfection, UV provides effective and rapid inactivation of microorganisms through a physical process. Inactivation by UV light act through the direct absorption of UV energy by the microorganism, causing a molecular rearrangement of one or more of the biochemical components that are essential to the organism's functioning. Microorganisms are inactivated by UV light as a result of damage to nucleic acids. The high energy associated with short wavelength UV energy, primarily at 254 nm, is absorbed by cellular RNA and DNA, this absorption forms new bonds between adjacent nucleotides, creating double bonds or dimers. Dimerization of adjacent molecules, particularly thymine, represents most common photochemical damage. Formation of thymine dimers in the DNA of viruses and bacteria prevents replication and inability to infect. UV light demonstrate efficacy against pathogenic organisms, including those responsible for typhoid, hepatitis, cholera, polio and other viral, bacterial and parasitic diseases [11]. Benefits of UV:

- UV produces no residual
- UV requires no transportation, storage or handling of toxic or corrosive chemicals – a safety benefit for plant operators and the surrounding community
- UV treatment creates no carcinogenic disinfection by-products that could adversely affect quality of the water
- UV is highly effective at inactivating a broad range of microorganisms – including chlorine-resistant pathogens like *Cryptosporidium* and *Giardia*
- UV can be used (alone or in conjunction with hydrogen peroxide) to break down toxic chemical contaminants while simultaneously disinfecting.

UV offers a key advantage over chlorine-based disinfection, due to its ability to inactivate protozoa that threaten public health – most notably *Cryptosporidium* and *Giardia.* The release of these harmful microorganisms into lakes and rivers by wastewater facilities utilizing chlorine disinfection increases the potential of contamination in communities that rely on these same bodies of water for their drinking water source and recreational use. Drinking water treatment plants can benefit by using UV since it can easily inactivate chlorine-resistant pathogens (protozoa), while reducing chlorine usage and by-product formation [43]. In addition, UV light, either alone or in conjunction with hydrogen peroxide can destroy chemical contaminants such as industrial solvents, pesticides and pharmaceuticals through a UV-oxidation [11]. Safety is a major concern since UV radiation can cause severe eye damage and skin irritation of exposed individuals. Furthermore, bacterial regrowth may occur because there is no residual antimicrobial activity. When exposed to visible light, bacterial cells that had been injured by UV light can repair themselves [44].

2.5.2 Ozone disinfection

Ozone is a very powerful disinfectant, unstable gas that can destroy bacteria and viruses. Is one of the strongest oxidation agents. It is an air pollutant of much concern in Europe, because it can affect human health and damage the environment. Because of its short half-life, ozone decay soon when produced. The half life of ozone in water is about 30 min, which means that every half hour the ozone concentration is reduced to half its initial concentration. In practice the half-life is shorter because a lot of factors (temperature, pH and concentration) can influence the half-life. Because ozone reacts with all kinds of components, the concentration ozone reduces quickly. The word ozone, from the Greek "*ozein*" [43], was first used in 1840 by the chemist C. F. Schonbein [45, 46], a professor at the University of Basel who sensed that, by subjecting oxygen to electric shock, a strange smell was emitted into the air, due to the presence of a gas called ozone. Ozone is a more effective disinfectant than chloramines, chlorine, and chlorine dioxide. Several studies proved that ozone, unlike chlorine products, can deactivate resistant micro-organisms. Although chlorine is very suitable for the deactivation of bacteria and viruses, it cannot be used to deactivate protozoa. Protozoa spread through the environment rapidly as cysts, which live longer and are more resistant to disinfectants than bacteria or viruses. In general, *Cryptosporidium parvum* causes larger problems for drinking water treatment than *Giardia Lambia* does. *Cryptosporidium parvum* is 4–5 μm in size, which makes it difficult to remove by conventional filtration [47]. *Giardia Lambia* is 8–14 μm in size, which makes it easier to remove by conventional filtration than *Cryptosporidium parvum* [17]. Moreover, when drinking water or swimming pool water is treated by means of conventional chlorination, *Cryptosporidium parvum* is insufficiently deactivated. Alternative treatment methods, such as ozone and UV disinfection, appear to have the ability to deactivate the oocysts sufficiently [33, 48]. The benefit of ozone is that it influences temperature and pH minimally on a broad spectrum. Ozone solubility decreases when temperatures rises, disinfection rates increase per 10°C. Within the range of 0–30°C, these two factors diminish one another. The disinfection rate of ozone hardly changes in a pH range of 6–8.5 [49]. For certain resistant microorganisms (such as *Giardia Muris*), the disinfection rate increases at higher pH values [10, 34], but for other species of microorganisms, this is the other way around. Other benefits of ozone application are:

- No remaining tastes or odors after treatment.
- Disinfection byproduct formation is minimal.
- Ozone can remove disinfection byproduct precursors.

Ozone is not always the most suitable disinfectant. Ozone is less suitable for maintenance of a residual concentration, causing it to decompose in water relatively quickly [49]. Chlorine is more suitable for residue formation [10].

2.5.3 Ultrasound

Ultrasound refers to inaudible sound waves with frequencies in the range of 16 kHz–500 MHz, greater than the upper limit of human hearing. It can be transmitted through any elastic medium including water, gas-saturated water, and slurry. Ultrasound has been used for diverse purposesin many different areas. In water treatment technology, the application of ultrasound (ultrasonication) can be useful in various processes like organic decontamination, disinfection, electrocoagulation, and membrane filtration. Because of cavitation phenomenon, the formation of free radicals and high localized temperatures and pressures, ultrasonic irradiation (ultrasonication) appears to be an effective method for the destruction of hazardous organic compoundsin water [50]. These compounds include phenol [51] chlorophenols, nitrophenols, aniline [52], trichloroethylene [53], ethylbenzene [54], chlorobenzene [55], chloronaphthalene, polychlorinated biphenyls, pesticides, polycyclic aromatic hydrocarbons, azobenzene, textile dyes [56], carbofuran, nitroaromatics, detergents and surfactants [57]. High power ultrasound, operatedat low frequencies is an effective means for disintegration of bacterial cells. However, disinfection by ultrasonication alone requires very high energy. Thus, generally it cannot be considered as an alternative to conventional disinfection for economical aspects. Then, ultrasonication should be used together with other techniques. For instance, the combination of a short ultrasonication and a subsequent ultraviolet treatment is even cost-efficient and meaningful [58]. Ultrasonication combined with chlorination improved significantly the biocidal action. These results suggest that ultrasound could be used in conjunction with chemical treatments to achieve a reduction in the quantity of bactericide required for water treatment [59]. Ultrasound irradiation can provide enhancement in membrane filtration of waste waters [60]. It increases the flux primarily by breaking the cake layer at the membrane surface. Liquid jets produced by cavitation served as a basis for ultrasonic membrane cleaning. Lower ultrasound frequencies have higher cleaning efficiencies than higher frequencies [61]. Intermittent ultrasound ir-radiation resulted in the same flux obtained as continuous irradiation but intermittent ultrasound consumed less energy and prolonged the lifetime of the membranes used, thus can be considered as a cost effective method of membrane cleaning [48]. Ultrasound can produce various effects on biological materials, for example, stimulating enzyme activity, cell growth, biosynthesis, etc., which enhances the bioactivity of the activated sludge. Thus, the improvement in efficiency of enhanced biological removal of phosphorus [62] and nitrogen [63]. Low frequency (25 kHz) was more effective than higher ones (80 and 150 kHz), or in other term, higher energy ultrasound was more efficient than lower energy ultrasound for the sludge treatment, indicating that mechanical effects, instead of free radicals, were responsible for the bioactivity enhancement [63]. Comparing with other pre-treatment methods, ultrasonication exhibits a great potential of not being hazardous to environment and for being economically competitive [64]. Ultrasound is used in the remediation of contaminated soil and sediment [47]. Ultrasonic leaching has been investigated for the decontamination of different types of soils from landfills, mining spills, and river sediments aswell as various types of contaminants like organic compounds. The application of ultrasound in air pollution control is based on acoustic agglomeration phenomenon that makes small particles precipitated for easy removal. Acoustic agglomeration is a process in which high intensity sound waves produce relative motion and collisions among fine particles suspended in gaseous media. Acoustic agglomeration can be conducted in two approaches, with low frequency and high frequency (ultrasound) sonication. While low frequency acoustic field is more cost and energy efficient, high frequency acoustic (ultrasonic) agglomeration might achieve better particle retention efficiency, especially for very small particles in submicron range [49].

3. Conclusion

Almost every environment on the planet contains microorganisms. Sanitation represents an applied science because of its importance to the protection of human health and its relationship with environmental factors that relate to health. This applied science relates to control of the biological, chemical, and physical hazards in a environment. Effective sanitation practices are needed to combat their proliferation and activity. Appropriate choice of disinfectant, setting clear goals and a reliable action plan are necessary steps to ensure the safety of animals, people, equipment and the environment.

Acknowledgements

The work was supported by the project VEGA 2/0125/17.

Conflict of interest

The authors declare no conflict of interest.

Abbreviations

pH	potential of hydrogen
HLD	high-level disinfectants
EPA	environmental protection agency
HIV	human immunodeficiency virus
OH^-	hydroxide ions
CO2	carbon dioxide
%	percentage
°C	degree Celsius
NaOH	sodium hydroxide
CaOH	calcium hydroxide
H^+	hydrogen ions
HCl	hydrochloric acid
HNO_3	nitric acid
H_3PO_4	phosphoric acid
CH_3COOH	peracetic acid
ml m^{-3}	milliliter per cubic meter
ClO^-	hypochlorite
PAL	surface active substances
UV	ultraviolet
nm	nanometer
RNA	ribonucleic acid
DNA	deoxyribonucleic acid
kHz	kilohertz
MHz	megahertz
EPA	environmental protection agency
EPS	extracellular polymeric substances
QS	quorum sensing

Author details

Mária Vargová[1*], Katarína Veszelits Laktičová[1], Rudolf Hromada[1], Iveta Cimboláková[2], Ivan Uher[2], Ingrid Papajová[3] and Korim Peter[1]

1 Department of the Environment, Veterinary Legislation and Economy, University of Veterinary Medicine and Pharmacy, Kosice, Slovak Republic

2 Pavol Jozef Safarik University in Kosice, Slovak Republic

3 Institute of Parasitology, Slovak Academy of Sciences, Kosice, Slovakia

*Address all correspondence to: maria.vargova@uvlf.sk

References

[1] Available from: https://www.npz.sk/sites/npz/Stranky/NpzArticles/2013_06/Zivotne_prostredie_a_jeho_vplyv_na_zdravie_cloveka.aspx?did=2&sdid=59&tuid=19&

[2] Available from: https://www.ciriscience.org/a_84-Principles-of-Cleaning-and-Disinfecting-Environmental-Surfaces

[3] Available from: https://www.svps.sk/potraviny/otazky.asp

[4] Available from: https://www.who.int/topics/foodborne_diseases/en/

[5] Mellor JE, Levy K, Zimmerman J, Elliot M, Bartram J, Carlton E. Planning for climate change: The need for mechanistic systems-based approaches to study climate change impacts on diarrheal diseases. The Science of the Total Environment. 2016;**548**:82-90. DOI: 10.1016/j.scitotenv.2015.12.087.s

[6] Favero MS, Bond WW. Chemical disinfection of medical and surgical materials. In: Block SS, editor. Disinfection, Sterilization and Preservation. 4th ed. Philadelphia: Lea & Febiger; 1996. pp. 17-41

[7] Dvorak G. Disinfection 101. Iowa State University: The Center for Food Security and Public Health; 2005

[8] VJC F. Disinfection of livestock production premises. Revue scientifique et technique (International Office of Epizootics). 1995;**14**(1):191-205

[9] Ondrašovič M, Ondrašovičová O, Sasáková N, Hromada R, Veszelits Laktičová K, Venglovský J, et al. Ochrana životného prostredia a verejného zdravia. Košice: UVLF; 2013

[10] Ondrasovic M, Ondrasovicova O, Vargova M, Kocisova A. Environmental Problems in Veterinary Practice. Kosice; 1997. p. 142. ISBN: 80-88867-15-0

[11] Štefkovičová M. Dezinfekcia a sterilizácia, teória a prax II. Žilina; 2007. pp. 88-90. ISBN: 978-80-968243-3-0

[12] Gilbert P, Allison DG, Mcbain AJ. Biofilms in vitro and in vivo: Do singular mechanisms imply cross-resistance? Journal of Applied Microbiology. 2002;**92**(Suppl):1-13

[13] Davey ME, Duncan MJ. Enhanced biofilm formation and loss of capsule synthesis: Deletion of a putative glycosyltransferase in *Porphyromonas gingivalis*. Journal of Bacteriology. 2006;**188**(15):5510-5523

[14] Carpentier B, Cerf O. Biofilms and their consequences, with particular references to hygiene in the food industry. Journal of Applied Bacteriology. 1993;**75**:499-511

[15] Wang HH, Meredith AME, Blaschek HP. Biofilms in the Food Environment. Iowa: Iowa State University Press; 2007. pp. 7-15. ISBN: 978-0813820583

[16] Available from: http://mansfield.osu.edu/~sabedon/black12.htm

[17] McDonnell G, Russell D. Activity, action and resistance. Clinical Microbiology Reviews. 1999;**17**(1):147-179

[18] Mandell GL, Bennet JE, Dolin R. Principles and Practice of Infectious Diseases. New York: Churchill Livingstone; 1995. pp. 19-21

[19] Petersen CHA, Dvorak GD, Spickler AR. Maddie's Infection Control Manual for Animal Shelters for Veterinary Personnel. 1st ed. Iowa: Iowa State University; 2008. ISBN: 0-9745525-7-7

[20] Available from: https://www.nycoproducts.com/resources/blog/types-of-disinfectants-how-to-make-the-best-choice-for-your-facility/

[21] McDonnell G. Antisepsis, Disinfection and Sterilization. Types, Action, and Resistance. Washington DS: ASM Press; 2007. pp. 79-140. ISBN: 978-1-55581-392-5

[22] Russell AD, Hugo WB. Chemical disinfectants. In: Disinfection in Veterinary and Farm Animal Practice. Oxford: Blackwell Scientific Publications; 1987. pp. 20-23

[23] Jeffrey DJ. Chemicals used as disinfectants: Active ingredients and enhancing additives. Revue scientifique et technique (International Office of Epizootics). 1995;**14**:57-74

[24] Beňo V, Para Ľ, Ondrašovičová O. Ochrana životného prostredia zoohygieny. Magnus: Košice; 1992. pp. 139-154

[25] Maris P. Modes of action of disinfectants. Revue scientifique et technique (International Office of Epizootics). 1995;**14**:47-55

[26] Seymour SB. Disinfection, Sterilisation and Preservation. Philadelphia: Lea & Febiger; 1983. pp. 717-750

[27] Block SS. Disinfection, Sterilization and Preservation. 5th ed. Philadelphia: Lippincott Williams & Wilkins; 2000. ISBN: 0-683-30740-11

[28] Ondrašovičová O, Vargová M, Ondrašovič M, Biswencel H, Kašková A, Nagy J. Sanitácia v mäso spracujúcich prevádzkach. In: Sborník referátú ze semináře o údržnosti masa. Skaský Dvůr; 2003. pp. 51-55

[29] Ondrašovič M, Ondrašovičová O, Bis-Wencel H, Toropila M, Krajňák M, Novák P, et al. Dezinfekcia v potravinárskom priemysle pri využití Persterilu. Brno: Ochrana zvířat a welfare; 2000. pp. 187-190. ISBN: 80-7305-386-1

[30] Available from: https://www.cdc.gov/infectioncontrol/guidelines/disinfection/disinfection-methods/index.html

[31] Kennedy J, Bek J, Griffin D. Selection and Use of Disinfectants. Lincoln: University of Nebraska Cooperative Extension G00-1410-A; 2000

[32] Grooms D. Biosecurity Guide for Livestock Farm Visits. Michigan: Michigan State University Extension Bulletin; 2003. p. E2842

[33] Mokgatla RM, Gouws PA, Brozel VS. Mechanisms contributing to hypochlorous acid resistance of a salmonella isolate from a poultry processing plant. Journal of Applied Microbiology. 2002;**92**(3):566-573

[34] Payment P. Poor efficacy of residual chlorine disinfectant on drinking water to inactivate waterborne pathogenes in distribution systems. Canadian Journal of Microbiology. 1999;**45**:709-715

[35] Rodgers JD, Cullagh JJ, Namee PT, Smyth JA, Ball HJ. An investigation into the efficacy of hatchery disinfectants against strains of staphylococcus aureus associated with the poultry industry. Veterinary Microbiology. 2001;**82**:131-140

[36] Fu E, McCue K, Boesenberg D. Chemical Disinfection of Hard Surfaces – Household, Industrial and Institutional Settings. Amsterdam: Elsevier Science; 2007. pp. 573-592. ISBN: 978-0-444-51664-0

[37] Springthorpa S, Sander M, Nolan K, Sattar SA, Morris R, Jofre J. Comparison of static and dynamic disinfection models for bacteria and viruses on water

of varying quality. Water Science and Technology. 2001;**43**:147-154

[38] Ewart SL. Disinfectants and control of environmental contamination. In: Smith BL, editor. Large Animal Internal Medicine: Diseases of Horses Cattle, Sheep and Goats. 3rd ed. St. Louis: Mosby; 2001. pp. 1371-1380

[39] Morley PS. Biosecurity of veterinary practices. Veterinary Clinics: Food Animal Practice. 2002;**18**:133-155

[40] Quinn PJ, Markey BK. Disinfection and disease prevention in veterinary medicine. In: Block SS, editor. Disinfection, Sterilization and Preservation. 5th ed. Philadelphia: Lippincott, Williams & Wilkins; 2001. pp. 1069-1103

[41] Gupta AK, Ahmad I, Summerbell RC. Fungicidal activities of commonly used disinfectants and antifugal phatmaceutical spray preparatyions against clinical strains of Aspergillus and Candida species. Medical Mycology. 2002;**40**:201-208

[42] Bjorland J, Sunde M, Waage S. Plasmid-borne smr gene causes resistance to quarterny ammonium compounds in bovine Staphylococcus aureus. Journal of Clinical Microbiology. 2001;**39**:3999-4004

[43] Available from: https://www.trojanuv.com/uv-basics

[44] Bojkov RD. International Ozone Commission: History and Activities. Bavaria, Germany: IAMAS Publication Series; 2012

[45] Bojkov RD. Surface ozone during the second half of the nineteenth century. Journal of Applied Meteorology and Climatology. 1986;**25**:343-352

[46] Rubin MB. The history of ozone. The Schönbein period. 1839-1868. Bulletin for the History of Chemistry. 2001;**26**:0-56

[47] Collings AF, Farmer AD, Gwan PB, Sosa Pintos AP, Leo CJ. Processing contaminated soils and sediments by high power ultrasound. Minerals Engineering. 2006;**19**:450-453. DOI: 10.1016/j.mineng.2005.07.014

[48] Muthukumaran S, Kentish S, Lalchandani S, Ashokkumar M, Mawson R, Stevens GW, et al. The optimization of ultrasonic cleaning procedures for dairy fouled ultrafiltration membranes. Ultrasonics Sonochemistry. 2005;**12**:29-35. DOI: 10.1016/j.ultsonch.2004.05.007

[49] Hoffmann TL. Environmental implications of acoustic aero-sol agglomeration. Ultrasonics. 2000;**38**:353-357. DOI: 10.1016/S0041-624X(99)00184-5

[50] Joseph JM, Destaillats H, Hung H, Hoffmann MR. The sonochemical degradation of azobenzene and related azodyes: Rate enhancement via Fenton's reactions. The Journal of Physical Chemistry A. 2000;**104**:301-307. DOI: 10.1021/jp992354

[51] Entezari MH, Petrier C, Devidal P. Sonochemical degradation of phenol in water: A comparison of classical equipment with a new cylindrical reactor. Ultrasonics Sonochemistry. 2003;**10**:103-108. DOI: 10.1016/S1350-4177(02)00136-0

[52] Goskonda S, Catallo WJ, Junk T. Sonochemical degradation of aromatic organic pollutants. Waste Management. 2002;**22**:351-356

[53] Drijvers D, Baets RD, Visscher AD, Langenhove HV. Sonolysis of trichloroethylene in aqueous solution: Vola-tile organic intermediates. Ultrasonics Sonochemistry. 1996;**3**:83-90. DOI: 10.1016/1350-1477(96)00012-3

[54] De Visscher AD, Van Langenhove HV, Van Eenoo PV. Sonochemical degradation of ethylbenzene in aqueous solution: A product study. Ultrasonics Sonochemistry. 1997;**4**(2):145-151. DOI: 10.1016/S1350-4177(97)00017-5

[55] Dewulf J, Langenhove HV, Visscher AD, Sabbe S. Ultrasonic degradation of trichloroethylene and chlorobenzene atmicromolar concentration: Kinetics and modeling. Ultrasonics Sonochemistry. 2001;**8**:143-150. DOI: 10.1016/S1350-4177(00s)00031-6

[56] Tezcanli-Guyer G, Ince NH. Degradation and toxicityreduction of textile dyestuff by ultrasound. Ultrasonics Sonochemistry. 2003;**10**:235-240. DOI: 10.1016/S1350-4177(03)00089-0

[57] Belgiorno V, Rizzo L, Fatta D, Rocca CD, Lofrano G, Nikolaou A, et al. Review on endocrinedisrupting-emerging compounds in urban wastewater: Occurrence and removal by photocatalysis and ultrasonic irradiationfor wastewater reuse. Desalination. 2007;**215**:166-176. DOI: 10.1016/j.desal.2006.10.035

[58] Blume T, Neis U. Improved wastewater disinfection byultrasonic pre-treatment. Ultrasonics Sonochemistry. 2004;**11**:333-336. DOI: 10.1016/S1350-4177(03)00156-1

[59] Mason TJ. Sonochemistry and sonoprocessing: The link, thetrends and (probably) the future. Ultrasonics Sonochemistry. 2003;**10**:175-179. DOI: 10.1016/S1350-4177(03)00086-5

[60] Kyllönen H, Pirkonen P, Nystrom M. Membrane filtration enhanced by ultrasound a review. Desalination. 2005;**181**:319-335. DOI: 10.1016/j.desal.2005.06.003

[61] Lamminen MO, Walker HW, Weavers LK. Mechanisms and factors influencing the ultrasonic cleaning of particle-fouled ceramic membranes. Journal of Membrane Science. 2004;**237**:213-223. DOI: 10.1016/j.memsci.2004.02.031

[62] Xie B, Wang L, Liu H. Using low intensity ultrasound to improve the efficiency of biological phosphorus removal. Ultrasonics Sonochemistry. 2008;**15**:775-781. DOI: 10.1016/j.ultsonch

[63] Zhang P, Zhang G, Wang W. Ultrasonic treatment of biological sludge: Floc disintegration, cell lysis and inactivation. Bioresource Technology. 2007;**98**:207-210

[64] Maos T, Hong SY, Show KY, Tay JH, Lee DJ. Acomparison of ultrasound treatment on primary and secondary sludges. Water Science and Technology. 2004;**50**:91-97

Chapter 5

Immune Alteration Caused by Fibrous and Particulate Environmental Substances

Naoko Kumagai-Takei, Suni Lee, Kei Yoshitome, Nagisa Sada, Yasumitsu Nishimura and Takemi Otsuki

Abstract

Fibrous and particulate environmental substances such as asbestos fibers and silica particles cause not only lung fibrosis but also various health disturbances. Asbestos induce malignant tumors such as pleural mesothelioma and lung cancer. Silicosis patients exposed to silica particles show complications of various autoimmune diseases such as rheumatoid arthritis, systemic lupus erythematosus, systemic sclerosis, and antineutrophil cytoplasmic antibody (ANCA)-related vasculitis/nephritis. The causative alteration of immune cells exposed to these environmental substances may form baseline modification of human immune system not only localized pulmonary lesions, alteration of alveolar macrophages, and others but also general immune system and changes of function in effector, regulatory, and cytotoxic T cells and natural killer cells. In this review, both (localized and generalized) immune alterations caused by environmental fibrous and particulate substances are summarized and reported.

Keywords: immune alteration, silica, asbestos, immune cells, autoimmunity, antitumor immunity

1. Introduction

The typical lung disease caused by occupational and environmental substances is pneumoconiosis [1, 2]. The pneumoconiosis is defined as health impairment caused by inhalation of dusts and mainly involves the lung. The restrictive lung disease defined as lung fibrosis occurred. The two main typical pneumoconioses are silicosis (SIL) and asbestosis [1, 2].

SIL is induced by inhalation of silica particle, SiO_2. It is white and powder form substance and relatively light. Thus, these particles deposit to the middle to the upper lobes of the lung [3, 4]. The alveolar macrophages (AM) are responsible to recognize these particles as external danger signal [5, 6]. Then, inflammasome inside of AMs, as dendritic cells, begin to initial reaction to produce cytokines such as interleukin (IL)-1β. The fibroblasts are called in to these area and form collagen deposition. Radiologically, these depositions of collagens are recognized as small nodules [5–7]. Thereafter, these nodules sometimes grow up more than 1 cm diameter defined as large nodules. The pathological lesions then spread many pulmonary complications such as tuberculosis, tuberculous pleurisy, secondary pneumothorax, secondary bronchitis, and secondary bronchiectasis. In addition, lung cancer is also considered as complication of SIL [1, 2, 7].

The other typical pneumoconiosis is asbestosis [8, 9]. The asbestos is fibrous substance. The asbestos fibers are classified as serpentine group and amphibole group [10, 11]. The former consists of only chrysotile, and the latter includes five fibers, i.e., amosite, crocidolite, tremolite, anthophyllite, and actinolite. The serpentine is curly and the amphibole group is needle-like. These fibers are fibrous, so they are relatively heavy. Thus, the deposition occurred in the middle to lower lung lobes. Then, as similar to silica particles, the inflammasome in AM is starting reactions to form fibrosis [5–7]. The difference of form of fibrosis depends on fibers' length. Asbestos fibers possess more than 3 aspect ratio, and thus it is relatively long [10, 11]. Then, the collagen deposition also forms irregular and kind of linear pathology, not like nodules caused by silica particulate substances. Radiologically it is defined as irregular shadows and sometimes develops to honeycomb shadow [8, 9]. Even though doses are not higher to cause asbestosis and lung fibrosis, other asbestoses causing complications are known. These are pleural plaque (PP), benign pleural effusion, rounded atelectasis, and diffuse pleural thickening [12, 13]. In addition, the important complications are malignant tumor such as lung cancers and malignant mesotheliomas (MM). In addition, the report from the International Agency for Research on Cancer (IARC) shows possibility of relation between asbestos exposure and laryngeal, gastrointestinal, ovarian, and bile-duct cancers [14, 15].

The SIL patients often complicate with autoimmune diseases [7, 16]. Caplan syndrome which is defined as complicated rheumatoid arthritis (RA) with coal miner pneumoconiosis is well known and classical. Additionally, various epidemiological studies indicated the complications of various autoimmune diseases such as systemic sclerosis (SSc), systemic lupus erythematosus (SLE), and, more recently, antineutrophil cytoplasmic antibody (ANCA)-related vasculitis/nephritis [7, 17]. To consider the mechanisms of causing dysregulation of immune tolerance in SIL patients, the exposure to silica particles may affect to the human immune cells to form bases.

Since asbestos fibers are different physiologically with silica particles, asbestos is fibrous, not particulate, but asbestos fibers are the mineral silicate. Thus, chemically, fibers consist of SiO_2 and other elements such as iron, magnesium, and sodium. The carcinogenic activity of asbestos is considered dependent on iron contents [14–18]. Therefore, crocidolite ($Na_2Fe^{2+}{}_3Fe^{3+}{}_2Si_8O_{22}(OH)_2$) is considered to possess the strongest carcinogenic activity, and amosite ($Fe_7Si_8O_{22}(OH)_2$) is assumed the next [14–18]. However, even though chrysotile ($Mg_3(Si_2O_5)(OH)_4$) does not contain iron, this serpentine fiber is also considered as a carcinogenic substance. Although the carcinogenic activity is lower than crocidolite and amosite, chrysotile also cause cancers by its physical form to induce AMs as frustrated (not being able to digest as foreign danger material and produce reactive oxygen species (ROS) as free radicals) and contamination of amphibole fibers as natural mineral products [14, 18, 19]. As mentioned above, silica particles are assumed to influence the human immune system [7, 17].

As shown in **Figure 1**, silica particles and asbestos fibers affect various immune cells such as CD4+ helper T (Th) cells (responder T cells: Tresp), Th17, regulatory T cells (Treg), CD8+ cytotoxic T lymphocyte (CTL), and natural killer (NK) cells. In this review, the effects of silica or asbestos on Tresp, Treg, and Th17 are compared and summarized from our findings as well as reported literatures. Thus, regarding effects of asbestos on CTL [20], briefly, the proliferation and differentiation using mixed lymphocyte reaction (MLR) assay were inhibited, as well as using in vitro activation assay with chrysotile fibers or analyses of peripheral blood CTL derived from patients with PP and MM. As a result, in CTLs from asbestos-exposed

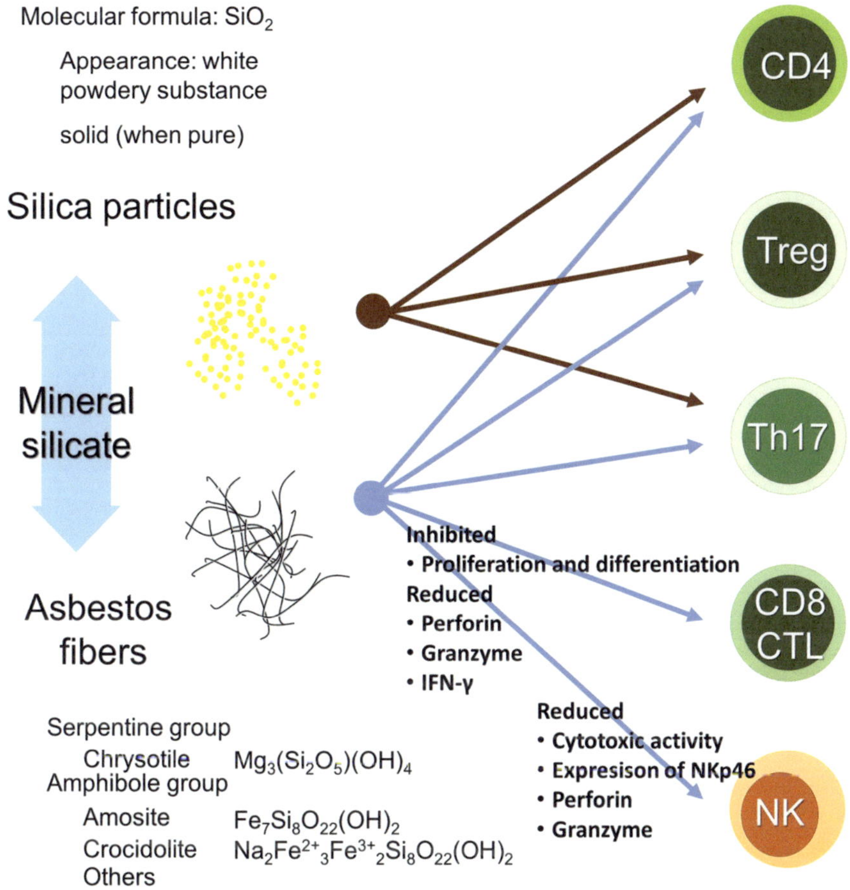

Figure 1.
The aim of this review is to present the effects of silica particles and asbestos fibers onto various human immune cells such as CD4+ T helper cell, regulatory T cell (Treg), Th17 cell, CD8+ cytotoxic T lymphocyte (CTL), and natural killer (NK) cell. Although physiological features of silica and asbestos are different, particulate and fibrous substances, chemically Si and O, are the core elements. For CTL, asbestos fibers inhibit its proliferation and differentiation as well as reduction of cytotoxic materials such as perforin, granzyme, and interferon (IFN)-γ. In addition, exposure to asbestos fibers on NK cell; its cytotoxic activity; expression of one of the activation receptors, NKp46; and production of cytotoxic molecules (perforin and granzyme) are reduced.

patients, especially in MM, cytotoxic molecules such as perforin, granzyme, and interferon (IFN)-γ were reduced. These results indicated that asbestos exposure causes reduction of antitumor immunity regarding CTL function [20–23].

In addition, in our analyses using NK cells derived from healthy volunteers (HV) and incubated with asbestos fibers, human NK cell line exposed to asbestos fibers continuously revealed some NK cell-activating receptors including NKG2D, NK2B4, and NKp46 and intracellular perforin and granzymes as shown in **Figure 1**. Particularly, the expression levels of NKp46 were correlated with NK cell killing activity against tumor cells. These results also indicated that asbestos exposure reduced antitumor immunity regarding NK cell function [24, 25].

2. Effects of silica particles and asbestos fibers on CD4+ Tresp

The effects of silica particles and asbestos fibers are shown in **Figure 2**.

Silica particles chronically activate Tresp cells. As a result, the expression of CD69, one of the earlier activating cell surface markers of Tresp, was gradually

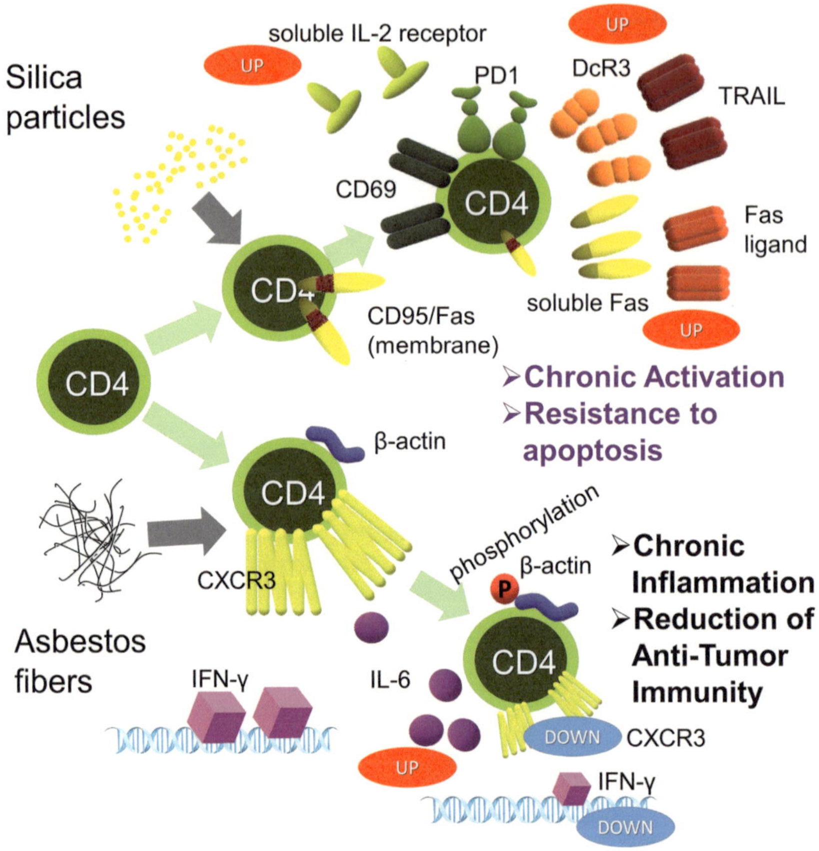

Figure 2.
The effects of silica and asbestos on CD4+ responder T cell. Silica caused chronic activation and resistance to Fas-mediated apoptosis. On the other hand, asbestos exposure causes chronic inflammation and reduction of antitumor immunity.

increased when peripheral blood mononuclear cells (PBMC) were incubated with silica in vitro [26]. In addition, the mRNA expression of program death-1 (PD-1) molecules as the activation marker of Tresp was compared between Tresp derived from HV and SIL patients. As a result, PD-1 was highly expressed in SIL than those in HV. Moreover, serum soluble IL-2 receptor (sIL-2R) concentration showed higher in SIL than HV [27]. The sIL-2R is considered as one of the markers which reveal chronic activation of Tresp, and various collagen diseases and autoimmune diseases are shown to be higher (not like T-cell tumors such as T-lineage malignant lymphoma and leukemias) than HV [28]. All of these results indicated that Tresp in SIL are chronically activated by silica exposure. It is assumed that circulating Tresp may repeat encounters with silica particles on lung fields and pulmonary lymph nodes [29].

On the other hand, serum from SIL showed higher soluble Fas (sFas) than these from HV [30]. The sFas is produced by alternative splicing of Fas, CD95, death receptor, and gene and binds with Fas ligand at the extracellular area. In addition, if sFas is alternatively spliced, transcription of original wild-type Fas is reduced. Thus, membrane Fas is decreased, and Fas ligands are consumed at the outer spaces [31]. Moreover, other spliced variants of Fas gene remained as binding site with Fas ligand and loose membrane-binding domain [32]. So, these may also act as sFas to prevent Fas ligand-induced apoptosis. In addition, similar scenario of sFas and Fas ligand is assumed in TNF-related apoptosis-inducing ligand (TRAIL) and its receptor. Similar to sFas, cells sometimes produce decoy receptor to TRAIL, such as membrane-bound decoy receptor (DcR) 1 and 2 and soluble DcR3 [33, 34]. In this viewpoint, mRNA of DcR3 was highly expressed in SIL PBMCs compared with those from HV [35]. In addition, serum DcR3 levels were also higher in SIL rather than HVs (data unpublished).

Taken together, Tresp exposed chronically and repeatedly to silica particles reveal chronic activation and resistance to apoptosis. Thus, chronically activated Tresp, in which probably self-antigen recognizing Tresp are also included, survive longer. This makes the chance of encounter Tresp and self-antigens more frequent [29, 36].

Regarding asbestos fibers, a human T-lymphotropic virus (HTLV) 1 immortalized human polyclonal T lymphocyte cell line, MT-2 [37], was applied to explore the chronic effects of asbestos on human T cells. Although temporally and relatively high-dose exposure induced ROS production, activation of mitochondrial apoptotic pathway, and cell death [38], relatively low-dose and continuous exposure (more than 8 months) in vitro afforded the acquisition of resistance to asbestos-induced apoptosis [39]. These continuously exposed sublines (exposed to chrysotile or crocidolite) revealed C-X-C chemokine receptor type (CXCR) 3 expression [40]. This receptor is important to call tumor-attacking T cells into the tumor surrounding area. In addition, one of the important cytokines against tumor cells, IFN-γ expression, was also decreased compared with asbestos-unexposed original cell line. These findings were confirmed using Tresp derived from PP or MM patients [41]. In addition, when Tresp derived from HV and patients with PP or MM were stimulated in vitro, IL-6 was produced higher in the supernatant of Tresp derived from PP or MM rather than those from HV [41].

In these findings together with the abovementioned asbestos' effects on CTL and NK cells, continuous asbestos exposure induces reduction of antitumor immunity and increases chronic inflammation [42]. These are assumed to be the one of the backgrounds for occurring mesothelioma after long latency since initial exposure to asbestos fibers and rapid progress of malignant tumor once it occurred [42].

Additionally, continuously exposed sublines showed excess phosphorylation of β-actin (**Figure 2**) with over binding of some molecules in cytoskeletal component such as vimentin, α-tubulin, and myosin 9 [43]. These indicate that changes of cytoskeletal molecules after continuous exposure to asbestos fibers possess important roles for alteration of cellular and molecular functions [43], since asbestos fibers are not adsorbed into the cell inside due to the fibers' size and physical properties.

3. Effects of silica particles and asbestos fibers on Treg

Treg is defined as CD4+, CD25+, and forkhead box P3 (FoxP3) as transcription factor positive [44]. Treg inhibit the activation and proliferation of Tresp after antigen stimulation. Thus, decreases of volume and function of Treg cause excess reaction to antigen including self-antigen. This proceeds to allergy and autoimmune diseases. Contrary, increases of function and volume of Treg suppress Tresp activation and proliferation. Thus, considering the complications in silica- or asbestos-exposed patients, the former show autoimmune disorders and the later present with malignant tumors. Therefore, silica may cause decrease of Treg's function or volume. On the other hand, asbestos may enhance Treg's function or volume [44–46].

Initially, Treg's (CD4+ and CD25+ fraction in PBMC derived from SIL) suppressive function against alloantigen-stimulated Tresp (CD4+ and CD25−) proliferation was assayed using MLR. As a result, Treg fraction from SIL was less suppressive than those from HV when added as one fourth to half of Tresp number [47]. Although this result indicated that silica exposure reduces the function of Treg, as mentioned above, Tresp in SIL were chronically activated to express CD25 on their cell surface as the activation. Thus, peripheral CD4+ and CD25+ fraction may include chronically activated Tresp. To confirm whether or not silica exposure reduces function of Treg or its volume, Fas expression in Treg (FoxP3+) between SIL and HV was compared, and those from SIL showed higher [27]. Thereafter, if PBMC from HV were cultured with silica particles in vitro, CD25-positive cells were increased in CD4+ cells, but FoxP3+ cells decreased [27]. The interpretation of this finding is that silica exposure induces chronic activation of Treg similar to Tresp. As a result, Treg express excess Fas and proceed to Fas-mediated apoptosis. Then, early loss of Treg occurred in the peripheral blood of SIL. Together with the abovementioned long survival and apoptosis resistance in Tresp from SIL, SIL showed an imbalance of Tresp and Treg (Tresp dominant), and this tendency is known in various autoimmune diseases (**Figure 3**). So, it can be considered that silica exposure yields the basic immune alteration which causes occurrence of autoimmune diseases [17, 48]. With some individual factors such as HLA types and other single-nucleotide polymorphisms (SNPs) in various genes related to immune function such as ILs or other growth factors such as TNF-α, SIL often complicates with autoimmune diseases.

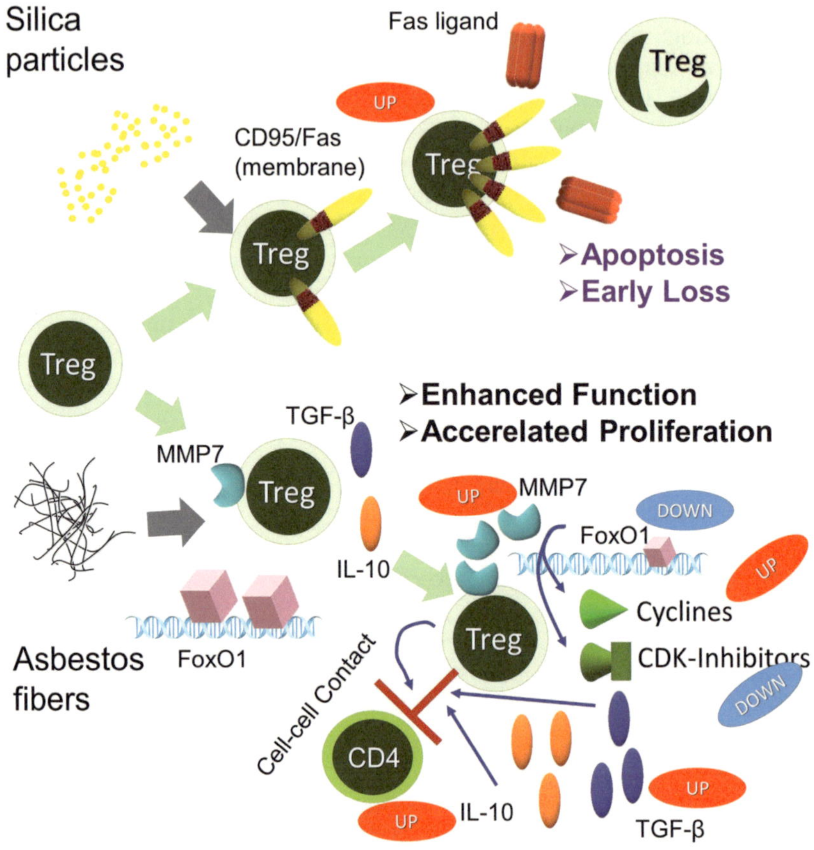

Figure 3.
The effects of silica and asbestos on Treg. Silica induces enhanced expression of death receptor, Fas, causing excess apoptosis and early loss of Treg. On the other hand, asbestos enhances Treg function via cell-cell contact and overproduction of soluble factors, IL-10 and TGF-β. In addition, asbestos-induced decreased expression of FocO1, transcription factor, causes acceleration of cell cycle progression by upregulation of cyclins and downregulation of CDK inhibitors. Taken together, asbestos induces enhancement of Treg quality and quantity causing reduction of antitumor immunity.

To investigate the effect of asbestos on Treg, the cell line, MT-2, which was used to continuous exposure model to asbestos, was reported to possess Treg-like function [49, 50]. Thus, the Treg function in original MT-2 cells which never meet with asbestos fibers and MT-2 subline continuously exposed to asbestos. As a result, inhibitory effects on Tresp proliferation were stronger in subline rather than original line by cell-cell contact assay. In addition, subline showed overproduction of IL-10 [39] and transforming growth factor (TGF)-β when compared with original line [51, 52]. Since these two cytokines are typical soluble factors for Treg suppressive function, knockdown clones for IL-10 or TGF-β were compared with their suppressive activity with subline using transmembrane assay (designing only soluble factors, but not cells, can slip through the membrane). As a result, Tresp proliferated much more with transmembrane cultured with knockdown clones for IL-10 or TGF-β than subline [51]. Thus, Treg function was enhanced by asbestos continuous exposure via cell-cell contact as well as excess production of soluble factors.

It was found that transcription factor, FoxO1, was reduced in asbestos' continuously exposed subline [53]. FoxO1 affects cell cycle regulator genes such as cyclins and cyclin-dependent kinase (CDK)-inhibitors (CDK-Is) such as ink4 family (p15, p16, p18, and p19) and cip/kip family ($p21^{cip1}$, $p27^{kip1}$, and $p57^{kip2}$). To compare the expression of cyclins and CDK-Is, cyclins were highly expressed, while CDK-Is were weakly expressed in subline compared with original cells. In addition, in cell cycle phase analysis, subline showed higher S/G1 ratio (S-phase% was divided with G1 phase%) than that of original line. In addition, knockdown of FoxO1 in subline using siRNA induced increased expression of cyclin D1, the most enhanced expression in subline [54]. These results indicated that reduced FoxO1 caused by asbestos exposure induced enhancement of cell cycle progression.

Taken together, asbestos exposure increases Treg function and volume (**Figure 3**).

In addition, it was found that matrix metalloproteinase (MMP)-7 gene expression was enhanced in asbestos-exposed subline rather than original line [55]. Although the role of this finding is not explored well, MMP-7 also known as matrilysin is considered as the enzyme related to the cancer metastasis and invasion to cut extracellular matrix such as proteoglycan, fibronectin, and collagen type IV [56]. In addition, MMP-7 affects apoptosis by cutting membrane-bound Fas ligand to proceed as soluble form. If Treg produce much more MMP-7 due to asbestos exposure, tumor-attacking Tresp may proceed to apoptosis. Although the detailed examinations should be done, this alteration may be important to consider asbestos exposure and tumor occurrence.

4. Effects of silica particles and asbestos fibers on Th17

Th17 cells are differentiated by cytokine balance surrounding T helper cells in balance with Treg. Th17 is promoted with IL-6 and TGF-β, whereas Treg is skewed only by TGF-β. Thus, this balance is important for both differentiations [57]. Th17 is considered to contribute to the occurrence of autoimmune diseases via cytokine production such as IL-17 and IL-22 [58]. Thus, it should be investigated how silica particles affect the function and volume of Th17 regarding complications of SIL. Unfortunately, there are no reports regarding this viewpoint. Future investigations are required to explore the role of silica particles on the function of TH17 and changes of volume.

On the other hand, there were couples of articles regarding Th17 and silica-induced lung fibrosis. Lo Re et al. reported that rapid lung recruitment of Th17 producing IL-17A was mediated by macrophage-derived IL-23 and was important to form inflammation, but not fibrosis, in experimental silicosis using animal model [59]. Then, Song et al. studied using mice model of silica-induced fibrosis and found Treg promotes Th17 differentiation via TGF-β1 and IL-1β [60]. Although they did not define inflammation and fibrosis in detail, there might be some role in Treg to activate Th17 for the development of lung fibrosis. Mills et al. found the importance of γδT cells with Th17 to produce IL-17 by analyzing details of inflammasome activation [61]. Thus, this study was not defined in silica-induced fibrosis. However, they considered the roles of Th17 and γδT cells for the development of many autoimmune and chronic inflammatory diseases. Thus, silica exposure may affect γδT cells, too. Chen et al. investigated that in the mouse model, neutralization of IL-17A delayed progression of silica-induced lung inflammation and fibrosis [62]. They assumed this was caused by decrease of IL-6 and IL-1β and increase of Treg. Song et al. from the same group showed the importance of IL-1β on lung fibrosis caused by silica using IL-1 type I receptor antagonist [63]. Then, their findings indicated that regulating IL-22 and IL-1β organizes Th1 and Treg differentiations, and then, these were important for promotion of lung inflammation caused by silica via Th17 promotion (**Figure 4**).

Interest reports to reveal importance of MyoD88 for lung fibrosis and inflammation caused by silica using MyD88 knockout mice were studied by Re et al. [64]. They found that accumulation of Treg and cytokines such as IL-10, TGF-β1, and platelet-derived growth factor (PDGF)-B contributed to lung inflammatory and granuloma responses, whereas this was not with Th17 influx. Furthermore, Dai et al. focused on the Wnt/β-catenin pathway for silica-induced fibrosis. They agreed with Th17 enhancement [65]. In addition, if they blocked Wnt/β-catenin pathway, Th1/Th2 polarization was delayed, and this delay was caused by Treg and Th2 response. Then, they suggested that Wnt/β-catenin pathway regulates Treg and contributes to fibrogenesis in silicosis. Additionally, other than Th17, Liu et al. reported the role of IL-10-producing regulatory B cell in silicosis, since this B cell increased in silica instillation in mouse model [66]. The produced IL-10 seemed to suppress Th1 response with IL-10 produced from Treg.

Back to Th17, Li et al. studied alteration of expression in 4-1BB (CD137, TNFRSF9) which is an inducible costimulatory receptor expressed on activated T cells, during lung injury caused by silica using animal model [67]. Then, inhibitor for 4-1BB revealed reduction of Th1 and Th17 responses measured by TNF-α, IFN-γ, and I-17A production. Thus, 4-1BB pathway is also involved in Th17 cells toward inducible lung fibrosis due to silica exposure.

Taken together, Th17 is assuming to possess an important role in silica-induced lung fibrosis via other immune cells such as Treg and γδT cells as well as various cytokines and signaling molecules.

How about the role of Th17 in asbestos-exposed pathology? Ferro et al. reported that amphibole, but not chrysotile, induced antinuclear autoantibodies (ANA) and IL-17 in mice model [68]. In this study, they also found that there was a significant increase of suppressor B cells defined by CD19+, CD5+, and CD1d+ in the lung as well as the spleen. They considered amphibole and serpentine groups can induce inflammatory change; however, only amphibole is able to yield an autoimmune response. In addition, their studies were extended to assess erionite, which is naturally occurring fibrous mineral and belongs to a group of minerals called zeolites, not asbestos [69]. Physically, this is resembling to amphibole. In addition, this fiber is known to be a human carcinogen. The prevalence of malignant pleural and peritoneal mesothelioma due to erionite exposure in the Cappadocia region of Central Anatolia, Turkey, is very high. Zebedeo et al. reported that exposure of erionite as well as amphibole asbestos on bone-marrow-derived macrophage caused increasing ANA positive prevalence

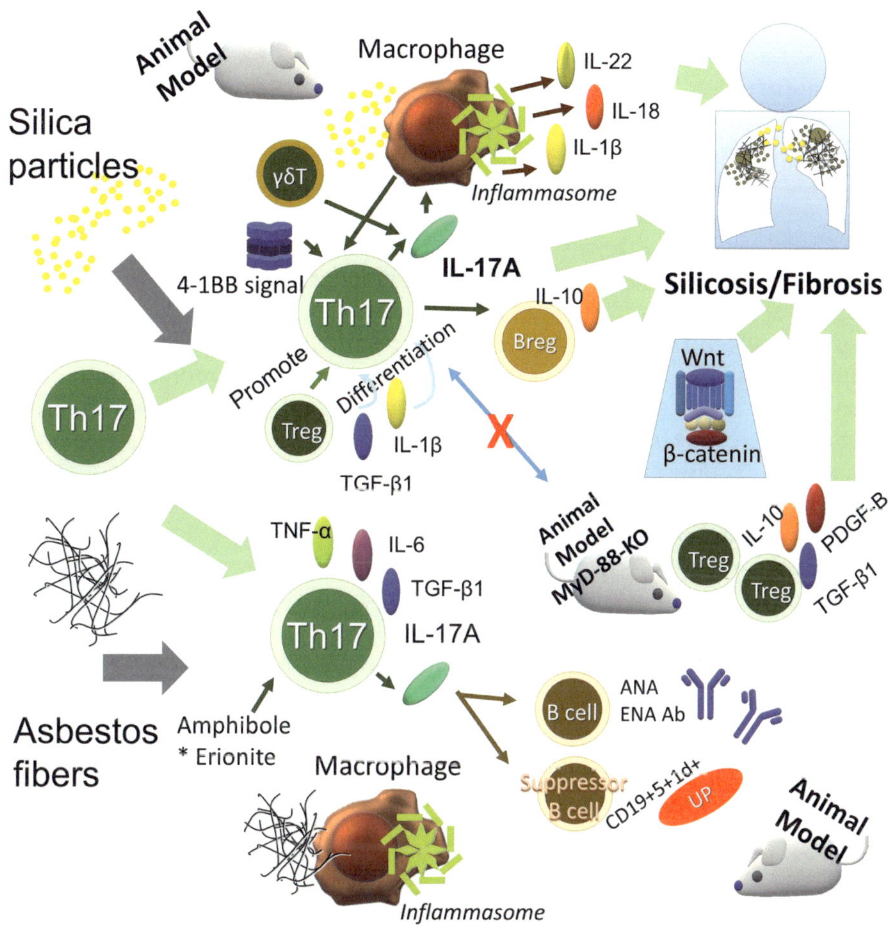

Figure 4.
Summarized effects of silica and asbestos from literatures on Th17 cell. Silica is related to the occurrence and development of lung fibrosis via Th17 cell with Treg and regulatory B cell. In addition, various molecules such as MyD-88, Wnt/β-catenin pathway, and 4-1BB signaling are also related with Th17 and silica-induced lung fibrosis. On the other hand, some reports showed amphibole asbestos and erionite affect Th17 cells to cause production of autoantibodies.

and elevation of serum concentrations of cytokines such as IL-17, I-6, TGFβ, and TNF-α [69]. Thus, they concluded that erionite and amphibole induce autoimmune dysregulation via Th17. Taken together, asbestos fibers may influence the Th17 and partially affect the occurrence of autoimmune diseases found in asbestos-exposed patients (**Figure 4**). However, the population of asbestos-induced autoimmune disease seems to be less than silica-exposed patients. Thus, further studies regarding individual factors and cellular and molecular mechanisms should be done.

5. Future overview

In this review, the immune effects of silica and asbestos are focused. Although exposure to silica particles and asbestos fibers is still an important issue in the world, recent concerns are immunotoxicity caused by exposure to nanomaterials. For example, Dhupal et al. reported that immunotoxicity of titanium dioxide nanoparticles [70] caused apoptosis via multiple Toll-like receptors and ROS-dependent mitogen-activated protein kinase (MAPK) pathway. Chen et al. reviewed immunotoxicity of silica nanoparticle [71]. They emphasized the importance of surfaces and shapes on silica nanoparticles to cause dysfunction, cytotoxicity, and genotoxicity. Calbiati et al. studied immunotoxicity caused by silver nanoparticles [72]. They found slight stimulation of pro-inflammatory cytokine production and humoral immune responses. Although various investigations regarding immunotoxicity induced by nanomaterials have been reported, what will be induced by continuous or recurrent low-dose exposure to these materials as well as combined exposure to various materials should be considered. To establish experimental models for these views seems to be difficult, because of difficulties to assess human examples for combined exposure for various materials.

Regarding silica and asbestos focused on this review, there may be combined exposure situation. Then, although we declared silica causes dysregulation of autoimmunity and asbestos induces reduction of antitumor immunity, how exposed individual people present which types of immunotoxicities is still difficult to predict. These may be dependent on individual factors such as human leukocyte antigen (HLA) typing and other genotyping such as various single-nucleotide polymorphisms (SNPs) in the immune-related genes and microenvironmental conditions inside the individual bodies.

In addition, with investigations of exposure to various materials using animal models and cell models using human- or animal-derived various immune cells, the comprehensive strategies to evaluate multiple views regarding combined and continuous exposures should be established in the future.

6. Conclusion

In this review, the effects of silica particles and asbestos fibers on human immune cells were summarized. Both silica and asbestos effects are not only defined in the pulmonary cells but also in immune cells. Especially, since silicosis patients are often complicated with autoimmune diseases, immune effects of silica seemed to regulate to form basic status of dysregulation of immune tolerance [17, 48]. However, regarding Th17, silica exposure is involved in silica-induced lung fibrosis, contrary to the studies regarding relationship between asbestos and Th17 which had been performed on the viewpoint of autoimmune dysregulation.

In another aspect, the effects of asbestos fibers on various human immune cells such as CTL, NK cells, Tresp, and Treg indicated that asbestos exposure reduced the antitumor immunity [55]. This may involve in tumor occurrences and rapid progression of asbestos-induced cancers such as malignant mesothelioma.

The typical lung disease caused by occupational and environmental substances is pneumoconiosis, silicosis, and asbestosis. However, both particulate and fibrous substances influence the human immune system to form lung fibrosis as well as immune disorders such as alteration of autoimmunity and/or antitumor immunity. To consider these findings, it may be possible to neutralize altered immune status in silica- or asbestos-exposed people to prevent the development of lung fibrosis as well as complicated autoimmune diseases of asbestos-induced cancers by taking some agents included in foods or physiologically active substances. Further studies to investigate these possibilities may support chemoprevention for particulate fibrous material-induced health disturbances.

Acknowledgements

The authors thank Ms. Tamayo Hatayama and Shoko Yamamoto for their valuable technical assistances.

Conflicts of interest

All authors declare that there are no conflicts of interest.

Author details

Naoko Kumagai-Takei[1], Suni Lee[1], Kei Yoshitome[1], Nagisa Sada[1,2], Yasumitsu Nishimura[1] and Takemi Otsuki[1*]

1 Department of Hygiene, Kawasaki Medical School, Kurashiki, Japan

2 Department of Biophysical Chemistry, Graduate School of Medicine, Dentistry and Pharmaceutical Sciences, Okayama University, Okayama, Japan

*Address all correspondence to: takemi@med.kawasaki-m.ac.jp

References

[1] Mandrioli D, Schlünssen V, Ádám B, Cohen RA, Colosio C, Chen W, et al. WHO/ILO work-related burden of disease and injury: Protocol for systematic reviews of occupational exposure to dusts and/or fibres and of the effect of occupational exposure to dusts and/or fibres on pneumoconiosis. Environment International. 2018;**119**:174-185. DOI: 10.1016/j.envint.2018.06.005

[2] Perlman DM, Maier LA. Occupational lung disease. The Medical Clinics of North America. 2019;**103**:535-548. DOI: 10.1016/j.mcna.2018.12.012

[3] McLoud TC. Occupational lung disease. Radiologic Clinics of North America. 1991;**29**:931-941

[4] Leung CC, Yu IT, Chen W. Silicosis. Lancet. 2012;**379**:2008-2018. DOI: 10.1016/S0140-6736(12)60235-9

[5] Luna-Gomes T, Santana PT, Coutinho-Silva R. Silica-induced inflammasome activation in macrophages: Role of ATP and P2X7 receptor. Immunobiology. 2015;**220**:1101-1106. DOI: 10.1016/j.imbio.2015.05.004

[6] Rabolli V, Lison D, Huaux F. The complex cascade of cellular events governing inflammasome activation and IL-1β processing in response to inhaled particles. Part Particle and Fibre Toxicology. 2016;**13**(40). DOI: 10.1186/s12989-016-0150-8

[7] Pollard KM. Silica, silicosis, and autoimmunity. Frontiers in Immunology. 2016;7(97). DOI: 10.3389/fimmu.2016.00097.

[8] Billings CG, Howard P. Asbestos exposure, lung cancer and asbestosis. Monaldi Archives for Chest Disease. 2000;**55**:151-156

[9] Ross RM. The clinical diagnosis of asbestosis in this century requires more than a chest radiograph. Chest. 2003;**124**:1120-1128

[10] Sporn TA. Mineralogy of asbestos. Recent Results in Cancer Research. 2011;**189**:1-11. DOI: 10.1007/978-3-642-10862-4_1

[11] Bandli BR, Gunter ME. A review of scientific literature examining the mining history, geology, mineralogy, and amphibole asbestos health effects of the rainy Creek igneous complex, Libby, Montana, USA. Inhalation Toxicology. 2006;**18**:949-962

[12] Lemen RA, Dement JM, Wagoner JK. Epidemiology of asbestos-related diseases. Environmental Health Perspectives. 1980;**34**:1-11

[13] Mossman BT, Gee JB. Asbestos-related diseases. The New England Journal of Medicine. 1989;**320**:1721-1730

[14] Albin M, Magnani C, Krstev S, Rapiti E, Shefer I. Asbestos and cancer: An overview of current trends in Europe. Environmental Health Perspectives. 1999;**107S2**:289-298

[15] Heintz NH, Janssen-Heininger YM, Mossman BT. Asbestos, lung cancers, and mesotheliomas: From molecular approaches to targeting tumor survival pathways. American Journal of Respiratory Cell and Molecular Biology. 2010;**42**:133-139. DOI: 10.1165/rcmb.2009-0206TR

[16] Steenland K, Goldsmith DF. Silica exposure and autoimmune diseases. American Journal of Industrial Medicine. 1995;**28**:603-608

[17] Lee S, Hayashi H, Mastuzaki H, Kumagai-Takei N, Otsuki T. Silicosis and autoimmunity. Current Opinion

in Allergy and Clinical Immunology. 2017;**17**:78-84. DOI: 10.1097/ACI.0000000000000350

[18] Liu G, Cheresh P, Kamp DW. Molecular basis of asbestos-induced lung disease. Annual Review of Pathology. 2013;**8**:161-187. DOI: 10.1146/annurev-pathol-020712-163942

[19] Toyokuni S. Iron addiction with ferroptosis-resistance in asbestos-induced mesothelial carcinogenesis: Toward the era of mesothelioma prevention. Free Radical Biology and Medicine. 2019;**133**:206-215. DOI: 10.1016/j.freeradbiomed.2018.10.401

[20] Kumagai-Takei N, Nishimura Y, Maeda M, Hayashi H, Matsuzaki H, Lee S, et al. Effect of asbestos exposure on differentiation of cytotoxic T lymphocytes in mixed lymphocyte reaction of human peripheral blood mononuclear cells. American Journal of Respiratory Cell and Molecular Biology. 2013;**49**:28-36. DOI: 10.1165/rcmb.2012-0134OC

[21] Kumagai-Takei N, Nishimura Y, Maeda M, Hayashi H, Matsuzaki H, Lee S, et al. Functional properties of CD8(+) lymphocytes in patients with pleural plaque and malignant mesothelioma. Journal of Immunology Research. 2014;**2014**:670140. DOI: 10.1155/2014/670140

[22] Kumagai-Takei N, Nishimura Y, Matsuzaki H, Lee S, Yoshitome K, Hayashi H, et al. The suppressed induction of human mature cytotoxic T lymphocytes caused by asbestos is not due to interleukin-2 insufficiency. Journal of Immunology Research. 2016;**2016**:7484872

[23] Kumagai-Takei N, Nishimura Y, Matsuzaki H, Lee S, Yoshitome K, Otsuki T. Decrease in intracellular perforin levels and IFN-γ production in human CD8+ T cell line following long-term exposure to asbestos fibers. Journal of Immunology Research. 2018;**2018**:4391731. DOI: 10.1155/2018/4391731

[24] Nishimura Y, Miura Y, Maeda M, Kumagai N, Murakami S, Hayashi H, et al. Impairment in cytotoxicity and expression of NK cell-activating receptors on human NK cells following exposure to asbestos fibers. International Journal of Immunopathology and Pharmacology. 2009;**22**:579-590

[25] Nishimura Y, Maeda M, Kumagai N, Hayashi H, Miura Y, Otsuki T. Decrease in phosphorylation of ERK following decreased expression of NK cell-activating receptors in human NK cell line exposed to asbestos. International Journal of Immunopathology and Pharmacology. 2009;**22**:879-888

[26] Wu P, Hyodoh F, Hatayama T, Sakaguchi H, Hatada S, Miura Y, et al. Induction of CD69 antigen expression in peripheral blood mononuclear cells on exposure to silica, but not by asbestos/chrysotile-A. Immunology Letters. 2005;**98**:145-152

[27] Hayashi H, Miura Y, Maeda M, Murakami S, Kumagai N, Nishimura Y, et al. Reductive alteration of the regulatory function of the CD4(+)CD25(+) T cell fraction in silicosis patients. International Journal of Immunopathology and Pharmacology. 2010;**23**:1099-1109

[28] Hayashi H, Maeda M, Murakami S, Kumagai N, Chen Y, Hatayama T, et al. Soluble interleukin-2 receptor as an indicator of immunological disturbance found in silicosis patients. International Journal of Immunopathology and Pharmacology. 2009;**22**:53-62

[29] Lee S, Hayashi H, Maeda M, Chen Y, Matsuzaki H, Takei-Kumagai N, et al. Environmental factors producing autoimmune dysregulation—Chronic activation of T cells caused by

silica exposure. Immunobiology. 2012;**217**:743-748. DOI: 10.1016/j.imbio.2011.12.009

[30] Tomokuni A, Aikoh T, Matsuki T, Isozaki Y, Otsuki T, Kita S, et al. Elevated soluble Fas/APO-1 (CD95) levels in silicosis patients without clinical symptoms of autoimmune diseases or malignant tumours. Clinical and Experimental Immunology. 1997;**110**:303-309

[31] Otsuki T, Sakaguchi H, Tomokuni A, Aikoh T, Matsuki T, Kawakami Y, et al. Soluble Fas mRNA is dominantly expressed in cases with silicosis. Immunology. 1998;**94**:258-262

[32] Otsuki T, Sakaguchi H, Tomokuni A, Aikoh T, Matsuki T, Isozaki Y, et al. Detection of alternatively spliced variant messages of Fas gene and mutational screening of Fas and Fas ligand coding regions in peripheral blood mononuclear cells derived from silicosis patients. Immunology Letters. 2000;**72**:137-143

[33] Golstein P. Cell death: TRAIL and its receptors. Current Biology. 1997;7:R750-R753

[34] Lin WW, Hsieh SL. Decoy receptor 3: A pleiotropic immunomodulator and biomarker for inflammatory diseases, autoimmune diseases and cancer. Biochemical Pharmacology. 2011;**81**:838-847. DOI: 10.1016/j.bcp.2011.01.011

[35] Otsuki T, Tomokuni A, Sakaguchi H, Aikoh T, Matsuki T, Isozaki Y, et al. Over-expression of the decoy receptor 3 (DcR3) gene in peripheral blood mononuclear cells (PBMC) derived from silicosis patients. Clinical and Experimental Immunology. 2000;**119**:323-327

[36] Otsuki T, Miura Y, Nishimura Y, Hyodoh F, Takata A, Kusaka M, et al. Alterations of Fas and Fas-related molecules in patients with silicosis. Experimental Biology and Medicine (Maywood, NJ). 2006;**231**:522-533

[37] Miyoshi I, Kubonishi I, Yoshimoto S, Shiraishi Y. A T-cell line derived from normal human cord leukocytes by co-culturing with human leukemic T-cells. Gan. 1981;**72**:978-981

[38] Hyodoh F, Takata-Tomokuni A, Miura Y, Sakaguchi H, Hatayama T, Hatada S, et al. Inhibitory effects of anti-oxidants on apoptosis of a human polyclonal T-cell line, MT-2, induced by an asbestos, chrysotile-A. Scandinavian Journal of Immunology. 2005;**61**:442-448

[39] Miura Y, Nishimura Y, Katsuyama H, Maeda M, Hayashi H, Dong M, et al. Involvement of IL-10 and Bcl-2 in resistance against an asbestos-induced apoptosis of T cells. Apoptosis. 2006;**11**:1825-1835

[40] Maeda M, Nishimura Y, Hayashi H, Kumagai N, Chen Y, Murakami S, et al. Reduction of CXC chemokine receptor 3 in an *in vitro* model of continuous exposure to asbestos in a human T-cell line, MT-2. American Journal of Respiratory Cell and Molecular Biology. 2011;**45**:470-479. DOI: 10.1165/rcmb.2010-0213OC

[41] Maeda M, Nishimura Y, Hayashi H, Kumagai N, Chen Y, Murakami S, et al. Decreased CXCR3 expression in CD4+ T cells exposed to asbestos or derived from asbestos-exposed patients. American Journal of Respiratory Cell and Molecular Biology. 2011;**45**:795-803. DOI: 10.1165/rcmb.2010-0435OC

[42] Matsuzaki H, Maeda M, Lee S, Nishimura Y, Kumagai-Takei N, Hayashi H, et al. Asbestos-induced cellular and molecular alteration of immunocompetent cells and their relationship with chronic inflammation and carcinogenesis. Journal of Biomedicine &

Biotechnology. 2012;**2012**:492608. DOI: 10.1155/2012/492608

[43] Maeda M, Chen Y, Kumagai-Takei N, Hayashi H, Matsuzaki H, Lee S, et al. Alteration of cytoskeletal molecules in a human T cell line caused by continuous exposure to chrysotile asbestos. Immunobiology. 2013;**218**:1184-1191. DOI: 10.1016/j.imbio.2013.04.007

[44] Gavin M, Rudensky A. Control of immune homeostasis by naturally arising regulatory CD4+ T cells. Current Opinion in Immunology. 2003;**15**:690-696

[45] Baecher-Allan C, Viglietta V, Hafler DA. Human CD4+CD25+ regulatory T cells. Seminars in Immunology. 2004;**16**:89-98

[46] Hori S, Sakaguchi S. Foxp3: A critical regulator of the development and function of regulatory T cells. Microbes and Infection. 2004;**6**:745-751

[47] Wu P, Miura Y, Hyodoh F, Nishimura Y, Hatayama T, Hatada S, et al. Reduced function of CD4+25+ regulatory T cell fraction in silicosis patients. International Journal of Immunopathology and Pharmacology. 2006;**19**:357-368

[48] Lee S, Matsuzaki H, Kumagai-Takei N, Yoshitome K, Maeda M, Chen Y, et al. Silica exposure and altered regulation of autoimmunity. Environmental Health and Preventive Medicine. 2014;**19**:322-329. DOI: 10.1007/s12199-014-0403-9

[49] Chen S, Ishii N, Ine S, Ikeda S, Fujimura T, Ndhlovu LC, et al. Regulatory T cell-like activity of Foxp3+ adult T cell leukemia cells. International Immunology. 2006;**18**:269-277

[50] Hamano R, Wu X, Wang Y, Oppenheim JJ, Chen X. Characterization of MT-2 cells as a human regulatory T cell-like cell line. Cellular & Molecular Immunology. 2015;**12**:780-782. DOI: 10.1038/cmi.2014.123

[51] Ying C, Maeda M, Nishimura Y, Kumagai-Takei N, Hayashi H, Matsuzaki H, et al. Enhancement of regulatory T cell-like suppressive function in MT-2 by long-term and low-dose exposure to asbestos. Toxicology. 2015;**338**:86-94. DOI: 10.1016/j.tox.2015.10.005

[52] Maeda M, Chen Y, Hayashi H, Kumagai-Takei N, Matsuzaki H, Lee S, et al. Chronic exposure to asbestos enhances TGF-β1 production in the human adult T cell leukemia virus-immortalized T cell line MT-2. International Journal of Oncology. 2014;**45**:2522-2532. DOI: 10.3892/ijo.2014.2682

[53] Matsuzaki H, Lee S, Maeda M, Kumagai-Takei N, Nishimura Y, Otsuki T. FoxO1 regulates apoptosis induced by asbestos in the MT-2 human T-cell line. Journal of Immunotoxicology. 2016;**13**:620-627. DOI: 10.3109/1547691X.2016.1143539

[54] Lee S, Matsuzaki H, Maeda M, Yamamoto S, Kumagai-Takei N, Hatayama T, et al. Accelerated cell cycle progression of human regulatory T cell-like cell line caused by continuous exposure to asbestos fibers. International Journal of Oncology. 2017;**50**:66-74. DOI: 10.3892/ijo.2016.3776

[55] Kumagai-Takei N, Yamamoto S, Lee S, Maeda M, Masuzzaki H, Sada N, Yu M, Yoshitome K, Nishimura Y, Otsuki T. Inflammatory alteration of human T cells exposed continuously to asbestos. International Journal of Molecular Sciences. 2018;19. pii: E504. doi: 10.3390/ijms19020504

[56] Ii M, Yamamoto H, Adachi Y, Maruyama Y, Shinomura Y. Role of matrix metalloproteinase-7 (matrilysin) in human cancer invasion, apoptosis,

growth, and angiogenesis. Experimental Biology and Medicine (Maywood, N.J.). 2006;**231**:20-27

[57] Lee YK, Mukasa R, Hatton RD, Weaver CT. Developmental plasticity of Th17 and Treg cells. Current Opinion in Immunology. 2009;**21**:274-280. DOI: 10.1016/j.coi.2009.05.021

[58] Louten J, Boniface K, de Waal Malefyt R. Development and function of TH17 cells in health and disease. The Journal of Allergy and Clinical Immunology. 2009;**123**:1004-1011. DOI: 10.1016/j.jaci.2009.04.003

[59] Lo Re S, Dumoutier L, Couillin I, Van Vyve C, Yakoub Y, Uwambayinema F, et al. IL-17A-producing gammadelta T and Th17 lymphocytes mediate lung inflammation but not fibrosis in experimental silicosis. Journal of Immunology. 2010;**184**:6367-6377. DOI: 10.4049/jimmunol.0900459

[60] Song L, Weng D, Liu F, Chen Y, Li C, Dong L, et al. Tregs promote the differentiation of Th17 cells in silica-induced lung fibrosis in mice. PLoS One. 2012;**7**:e37286. DOI: 10.1371/journal.pone.0037286

[61] Mills KH, Dungan LS, Jones SA, Harris J. The role of inflammasome-derived IL-1 in driving IL-17 responses. Journal of Leukocyte Biology. 2013;**93**:489-497. DOI: 10.1189/jlb.1012543

[62] Chen Y, Li C, Weng D, Song L, Tang W, Dai W, et al. Neutralization of interleukin-17A delays progression of silica-induced lung inflammation and fibrosis in C57BL/6 mice. Toxicology and Applied Pharmacology. 2014;**275**:62-72. DOI: 10.1016/j.taap.2013.11.012

[63] Song L, Weng D, Dai W, Tang W, Chen S, Li C, et al. Th17 can regulate silica-induced lung inflammation through an IL-1β-dependent mechanism. Journal of Cellular and Molecular Medicine. 2014;**18**:1773-1784. DOI: 10.1111/jcmm.12341

[64] Re SL, Giordano G, Yakoub Y, Devosse R, Uwambayinema F, Couillin I, et al. Uncoupling between inflammatory and fibrotic responses to silica: Evidence from MyD88 knockout mice. PLoS One. 2014;**9**:e99383. DOI: 10.1371/journal.pone.0099383

[65] Dai W, Liu F, Li C, Lu Y, Lu X, Du S, et al. Blockade of Wnt/β-catenin pathway aggravated silica-induced lung inflammation through Tregs regulation on Th immune responses. Mediators of Inflammation. 2016;**2016**:6235614. DOI: 10.1155/2016/6235614.

[66] Liu F, Dai W, Li C, Lu X, Chen Y, Weng D, et al. Role of IL-10-producing regulatory B cells in modulating T-helper cell immune responses during silica-induced lung inflammation and fibrosis. Scientific Reports. 2016;**6**:28911. DOI: 10.1038/srep28911

[67] Li C, Du S, Lu Y, Lu X, Liu F, Chen Y, et al. Blocking the 4-1BB pathway ameliorates crystalline silica-induced lung inflammation and fibrosis in mice. Theranostics. 2016;**6**:2052-2067

[68] Ferro A, Zebedeo CN, Davis C, Ng KW, Pfau JC. Amphibole, but not chrysotile, asbestos induces anti-nuclear autoantibodies and IL-17 in C57BL/6 mice. Journal of Immunotoxicology. 2014;**11**:283-290. DOI: 10.3109/1547691X.2013.847510

[69] Zebedeo CN, Davis C, Peña C, Ng KW, Pfau JC. Erionite induces production of autoantibodies and IL-17 in C57BL/6 mice. Toxicology and Applied Pharmacology. 2014;**275**:257-264. DOI: 10.1016/j.taap.2014.01.018

[70] Dhupal M, Oh JM, Tripathy DR, Kim SK, Koh SB, Park KS.

Immunotoxicity of titanium dioxide nanoparticles via simultaneous induction of apoptosis and multiple toll-like receptors signaling through ROS-dependent SAPK/JNK and p38 MAPK activation. International Journal of Nanomedicine. 2018;**13**:6735-6750. DOI: 10.2147/IJN.S176087

[71] Chen L, Liu J, Zhang Y, Zhang G, Kang Y, Chen A, et al. The toxicity of silica nanoparticles to the immune system. Nanomedicine (London, England). 2018;**13**:1939-1962. DOI: 10.2217/nnm-2018-0076

[72] Galbiati V, Cornaghi L, Gianazza E, Potenza MA, Donetti E, Marinovich M, et al. *In vitro* assessment of silver nanoparticles immunotoxicity. Food and Chemical Toxicology. 2018;**112**:363-374. DOI: 10.1016/j.fct.2017.12.023

Chapter 6

Toward an Economic and Environmental Sustainability of the Health Systems of Western Countries

Andrés J. Ursa Herguedas

Abstract

One of the pillars of well-being, together with education and social coverage, is health. The various health systems currently existing in the world, both in advanced countries and in developing countries, do not comply with the principle of equity and, therefore, the Charter of Human Rights, by not universally covering the entire population. The great economic differences continue to feed off the poorest. The causes of mortality are still different between both worlds. The objective of this contribution is to sensitize political leaders at the international level, so that they adopt global agreements on the adequate use of energy, access to health and universal education to benefit the planet and its population. Integrative medicine, implemented in advanced and developing countries, with the use of conventional and unconventional treatments, the latter endorsed with scientific studies, has shown in recent decades that increases the preventive and curative possibilities, reduces the effects side effects of medication and contributes to environmental and economic sustainability. International health agencies should consider the proposal of incorporating integrative medicine into health systems and allocate financial resources to validate those techniques or procedures that do not yet enjoy scientific evidence. The population and political leaders must be sensitized by the state through which the planet Earth passes, in order to take large-scale measures to address socio-economic and environmental crises.

Keywords: welfare state, universal health, integrative medicine, environmental sustainability, climate change

1. Introduction

The pillars of well-being, centered on education, health and social achievements, have been a breakthrough in most developed countries. Faced with these real advantages, there is a series of uncertainties such as climate change, the instability of international politics that may be associated with an economic recession, the aging of the population and migratory flows, which threaten not only the stability of the system based on capitalism but the entire planet.

From the Industrial Revolution to the present day scientific and technical advances have contributed to social welfare, although there were many adverse political and economic scenarios to reach the current situation or according to the phrase of the Swiss economist Simonde de Sismondi "Production increases, while welfare decreases" [1].

The new industrial paradigm needed fossil fuels to be able to carry out all its activity. The traditional coal was introduced into oil and in the twentieth century nuclear energy. The "black gold" became one of the most precious assets on the planet, to the point of influencing the global economy and being able to cause wars. What has been produced for thousands of years in the terrestrial and marine subsoil, is consumed in a few decades, sends its combustion gases to the atmosphere, with the consequent environmental impact.

The reports on the production of energy by the fission of the atom were favorable for a good part of the scientific community. Disasters such as Chernobyl (Ukraine, 1986) and Fukushima (Japan, 2011), had to happen for politicians to reflect on and close the nuclear power plants in many countries.

In all these years there have been great advances in terms of food and nutrition. The progressive increase of the world population started speculation in food policy. Despite the intervention of international organizations such as the United Nations (UN) or the United Nations Food and Agriculture Organization (FAO), a good part of the population continues to go hungry, despite the abundance of food.

The overproduction of food to provide food to all the inhabitants of the planet goes through monocultures, the creation of transgenic products, the use of insecticides and chemical fertilizers. The earth is extracted more than what is entered. The literally dead earth is not able to withstand the torrents of water that are happening due to climate change and is carried by rivers to the sea [2]. Nutrients from plant-derived foods obtained intensively, as well as farm animals for human consumption, may not be as healthy as you would like them to be.

Many of the best fishing grounds of the entire planet have been overexploited and are on the verge of disappearing if no political measures are taken based on scientific reports [3]. Industrial and urban waste ends up in the sea, returning through the food chain to the humans themselves. Suffice it to mention the concentration of mercury and other heavy metals in the fish that occupy the top of the food chain or the microplastics found in fish extracted from the sea.

In recent decades there has been an increase in the number of diseases, at least in the West, with a high incidence of cancer [4] to the point that it is estimated that it will surpass cardiovascular diseases in the near future. There has been progress in the treatment of cancer, but not in prevention, so their numbers will continue to rise. The prevention of cancer is to adopt a healthy lifestyle, but this is not always enough if you live in a city contaminated by road traffic, noise, stress, etc.

The appearance of new diseases may be influenced and/or associated with the alteration of the natural environment produced by humans. It will be necessary to update the human pathology books and adapt the chapters to the new situation and create new ones if new diseases are described.

2. Health sciences at the service of humanity

2.1 From Hippocratic medicine to current health sciences

The considered "Father of medicine", Hippocrates, of the Greek island of Cos and his followers laid the foundations of current medicine, distinguishing between the magical-empirical and the scientific. Hippocratic doctors had the merit of considering medicine as a "technical" knowledge (ars medica) based on scientific knowledge of nature (physiology) [5]. In the Corpus Hippocraticum, set of the 53 anonymous writings, the Hellenic medical knowledge of the fifth century AC is collected, up to six centuries later [5]. In **Figure 1** you can see one of the representations of Hippocrates.

Of the diverse ancient cultures, the knowledge of the Egyptians on medicine, collected in the different papyri (Ebers, Smith, Hearst, etc.), dating from 1900 BC to 1200 BC [6].

In the East, the medicine of ancient Chinese, based on Taoism (see sign in **Figure 2**), considered the principles of yin and yang, as well as the elements water, earth, fire, wood and metal, as the basis of their preventive and therapeutic actions. They devised techniques such as acupuncture, moxibustion and various practices that have survived to this day. In the treatise Nei King, attributed to Emperor Huang Ti (2610 AC) the aspects about life and illness are collected [7].

We know about the medicine of ancient India for the texts that make up the Veda, which began to be written about the year 1500 AC. The Ayurvedic medical system distinguished seven organic elements, with a certain resemblance to the humors theory of hippocratism. The "traditional medicine" of India had as its common objective the unification of body-mind and spirit, proclaiming that disease and health would be the result of the confluence of three main aspects of existence (doshas) [8].

It is fair to highlight the ancient medicine of Japan, Israel and the pre-Columbian American, facing the corresponding cultural exchanges, with mutual influences, reflected in current medicine. The figure of Galen of Pergamum (131–203 AD) exerted great influence on medicine until well into the Middle Ages, with its successes and errors. He was able to transmit to the present day the theory of the humors of the Hippocratics [9].

Arab medicine from the East reaches a high level in the tenth and eleventh centuries, with talents such as Rhazes, author of numerous books and articles on philosophy, physics and medicine [10]. The great Avicenna (980–1037) left some 200 works, among others, with themes of medicine such as the Canon of medicine, with a discreet galenic influence [11].

In the twelfth and thirteenth centuries, with the expansion of Islam in the Iberian Peninsula include Avenzoar, Avempace and Averroes (1126–1198), the latter author of the Liber universalis de medicina [12]. The Jewish doctor Cordovan Maimonides (1135–1204) with his writings on toxicology, hygiene and deontology, made great contributions to the medicine of the time [13].

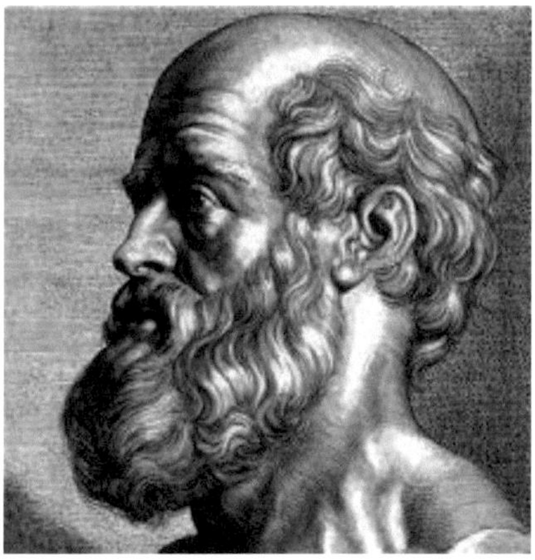

Figure 1.
Hippocrates.

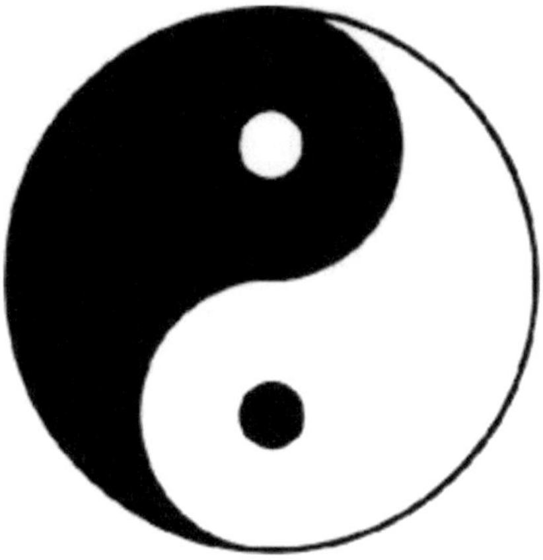

Figure 2.
Sign of Taoism.

Medieval European medicine survived, without major advances, thanks to the conservative work of the monasteries, hence the other name with which it is known (monastic medicine). The first universities are created, the monasteries are hospitals and it is the religious who provide care for the most disadvantaged. The first secular medical institution is created, the School of Salerno, near the current Naples (Italy). Founded in the ninth century, it reached its maximum splendor in the tenth and thirteenth centuries [14].

The School of Translators of Toledo (Spain) contributed to the knowledge of the Greek and Arab texts of Western Europe in the Middle Ages [15]. Throughout the thirteenth and fourteenth centuries, the universities of Bologna, Paris, Oxford, Salamanca, Cambridge, Naples, Padua, Vienna, etc. arose in Europe, with the "scholastic" method as a paradigm. The "black death" that decimated the European population since 1348 was also an important economic recession.

The history of medicine considers Arnau de Vilanova (1238–1311) as the most interesting character in medieval medicine. He worked as a doctor, clergyman and ambassador of kings and popes [16]. The dissection in human cadaver was an advance in anatomical science. The great discoveries in medicine begin with the circulation of blood by William Harvey (1578–1657). Cartesianism along with the thought of Galileo opens a new system in Medicine, iatromechanics. Its initiator, not doctor, Giovanni A. Borelli (1608–1679) introduced the mechanics applied to medicine [17].

In the Renaissance stand out the panvitalists Paracelso and van Helmont. The influence of the first in current medicine was decisive, so I highlight the most significant. Theophrastus Phillippus Aureolus Bombastus von Hohenheim, better known as Paracelsus (1493–1541), has gone down in history as a doctor ahead of his time. It contributed greatly to the fact that medicine followed a more scientific path and distanced itself from the theories of the scholastics. He began "specific" treatments and is considered the initiator of iatrochemistry [18].

Clinical medicine, as it is understood today, began in Padua in the sixteenth century and then spread to the rest of Europe. It was continued in Leiden (Kyper, Silvio, and Boerhaave), Vienna, Paris, London, etc., completed with necropsy later. Thomas Sydenham (1624–1689), considered one of the most prominent clinicians of all time, known as the "English Hippocrates," is the first to give name to diseases (morbid species). He distinguished acute diseases from chronic diseases and addressed the topic of the Hippocratic "epidemic constitution" with its own interpretation [19].

Vitalism as understood by Aristotle and the physicians of the seventeenth and eighteenth centuries with the "vital force" of Friedrich Kasimir Medikus (Von der Lebenskraft, 1774), breaks into this period of time in the medicine of the time [20]. In the eighteenth century, the first medical specialties began to appear. Thus, in 1787 there was already a specialized clinic for deliveries in Copenhagen [21]. Meanwhile, the clinical approach of medicine had been integrated with the anatomopathological one thanks to the publication and dissemination of the masterpiece by G. B. Morgagni [22].

At the doctrinal level, the ways of curing focus on the "contrary contrariis curantur" and "similia similibus curantur", both of which are stated in Hippocratic medicine. The principle of similarity was set in motion by the German physician Samuel F. Christian Hahnemann (1755–1843), creator of homeopathy. Homeopathy, more than a method, is considered as a general medical system [23] and is currently widely disseminated worldwide.

Due to the warlike conflicts numerous wounded ones took place, fact that served so that the surgery advanced. Weapon wounds and traumatic wounds gave way to gunshot wounds. One of the most prominent characters in this field was Ambroise Paré (1510–1590). Paré began his career as an apprentice surgeon-barber, a name by which a lower class of surgeons was known. The latter were below the so-called long-gown surgeons, who studied at the San Cosme School, knew the classical languages and writings of Galen. Barber surgeons were considered manual workers who, in addition to treating wounds, cut their hair, shaved and performed bloodletting. His contributions to the surgery on ligation of arteries, treatment of wounds by firearm, intrauteric turning of the child with breech presentation, and design of devices (trusses, etc.), made him be awarded the doctorate in medicine and out doctor of camera. He left several writings in the vernacular [24]. The Italian version of Paré was Bartolomeo Maggi (1516–1552), doctor of the pontifical army, who participated in the site of Mirandola with his colleague Giovanni Francesco Rota. His most important work is a treatise on gunshot wounds [25].

In the early sixteenth century sangria in Europe was still used, along with the purge, extending until the nineteenth century [26].

Dietetics, already initiated by the Hippocratics and continued by Galen, broke out in the sixteenth century with Lobera de Ávila, Luigi Cornaro, Tissot and Hufeland, the latter with his work Makrobiotic or art of prolonging life (1796) [27]. Hydrotherapy emerges enthusiastically in several European countries almost simultaneously, with the help of empiricists (Priesnitz, Kuhne, Kneipp, etc.) and doctors (Floyer, Hahn, etc.) [28]. Francois Magendi (1738–1855) founded in 1830 the first laboratory of experimental medical physiology in France. His disciple Claudius Bernard (1813–1878) surpassed his master by expressing his experiences in the book Introduction to the study of experimental medicine published in 1865. He has the concept of internal environment, which later would serve Haldane and Cannon to devise the term homeostasis [29]. The vaccines are preceded by Edward Jenner (1749–1823), with smallpox inoculation [30]. Medical Microbiology bases its findings on the findings of Pasteur (1822–1895), Lister (antisepsis) and Koch (1843–1910) [31]. At the same time, Immunology was developed with Metchnikoff (1884–1892), Ehrlich, etc. [32]. Biochemistry initiated in France is consolidated in Germany by Liebig (1803–1873) [33]. The X-rays are perfected and applied in the diagnosis from 1895 by Röntgen, assuming a breakthrough in the diagnosis of bone lesions [34].

At the end of the nineteenth century Wundt (1832–1920) inaugurated the first laboratory of experimental psychology in Leipzig (Germany). From here, several theories would emerge, some of them valid, to explain the psyche [35].

The advances in physics with Einstein, the spouses of Curie and Planck, to mention only the most significant, allowed to create the theoretical basis for the diagnostic and therapeutic advancement based on physics [36]. Genetics makes its appearance in the hands of Galton (1822–1911), Mendel (1822–1884) and Weismann (1834–1914) [37]. The start-up of the microscope, with its different variants, destroyed the fibrillar theory of past centuries and begins the era of cellular theory. In consonance with this is born the cellular pathology of Rudolph Virchow (1821–1902) [38].

2.2 The rise of pharmacological medicine

Although the Hippocratic doctors of the fourth century BC prescribed medicinal plants and some other potion, it was not until the emergence of the great doctors who exercised for the Roman Empire, which brought together the knowledge about the plant species applied in the medicine of the time. One of the most famous doctors in this regard was Dioscorides. Pedacio Dioscorides, born in Anazarbus, in Asia Minor, was a military surgeon of the Roman armies, in the time of Nero. He wrote "De Materia Medica" which served as a pharmacopeia manual until the Renaissance, this work being considered the forerunner of modern pharmacology [39].

During the Middle Ages, except for contributions from the Arab world, there were hardly any advances in therapy. Only the amanuenses of the monasteries, through copies of books, were the transmitters of medical knowledge. In 1085, the conquest of Toledo in Spain by Alfonso VI made it possible to combine ancient knowledge through the translation of classical texts. Through the collaboration of Arabs, Jews and Castilians, it was possible to translate philosophical, theological, astronomical, medical and other sciences texts into Spanish. Schools of translators were founded in Toledo, Seville and Murcia. The interpreters of countries like England, Germany and Italy took this knowledge to their respective countries, being an incentive for the foundation of several universities [40].

It would be necessary to reach the Renaissance with Paracelsus, the initiator of iatrochemistry, to advance in the treatment of diseases with chemical substances. The iatrochemistry, devoid of panvitalism and adapted to the mechanicism of the moment, survived until the seventeenth century. It is considered a precursor of current Pharmacology and Biochemistry [41]. Practically the treatment of diseases with plants with medicinal properties was one of the few options with which it was counted for centuries, apart from the knowledge about surgery that emerged. The term Phytotherapy was coined by Leclerc in 1913 [42]. In the university studies of Pharmacy is taught in Botany and Pharmacognosy, being important the number of investigations that are realized anywhere in the world in this matter.

In the first third of the twentieth century, as a result of the scientific-technical discoveries applied in the health sciences, new drugs are discovered that can cope with deadly and/or invalidating diseases such as certain infections. At first many of the drugs used came from the Plant Kingdom, such as the Salix genera where salicylic acid was obtained, alkaloids of the poppy (*Papaver somniferum*), digitalis obtained from various *Digitalis* species (*D. purpurea*, *D. lanata*, etc.), colchicine obtained from *Colchicum autumnale* used in the treatment of gout, etc., others were obtained from fungi and bacteria such as antibiotics. Later, in the course of the two major world races progress was made in surgery, pharmacology and radiotherapy. Currently most of the drugs are synthetic or are manufactured by genetically manipulated living beings.

Current medicine prevents, treats, restores, cures and rehabilitates numerous pathologies that were previously invalidating and/or fatal. Gone are many of the procedures that did not surpass the scientific method for their validation as the homeopathic system.

2.3 Medicine there is only one

"Medicine there is only one" is a phrase that has been devoted to time. The Spanish scientist José Miguel Mulet adds "and is effective when he has a scientific evidence behind it" [43].

Currently in the world much of the population does not have a health system that can meet the health needs of the inhabitants of that country, despite being a recognized right in the Universal Declaration of Human Rights (U.D.H.R, article 25.1). Many populations of the Third World must make use of the remedies offered by nature to deal with their diseases, using the experience transmitted for generations.

Although this inequality is not acceptable from the ethical point of view, it has a positive vision provided that nature is not frazzled, because they use local resources, with greater or lesser success, and do not use pharmacological remedies in the style of rich countries, which use many resources in their production, they are abused, they produce numerous secondary effects and many of them do not cure, maintaining the chronicity until advanced ages, with the consequent expense in human and material resources.

In many of the countries of the planet, integrative medicine is used, according to David Rakel, founder and director of the Department of Integrative Medicine at the University of Wisconsin (USA), "is oriented to the restitution of health and highlights the importance of the relationship between the doctor and the patient as a central aspect. It focuses on less invasive, less toxic and less expensive methods to try to facilitate health by integrating both conventional treatment modalities and complementary modalities. Its recommendations are based on an understanding of the physical, emotional, psychological and spiritual aspects of the human being" [44].

The World Health Organization, through its strategy on traditional medicine 2014–2023 of 2013 [45] and resolution WHA.67a of 2014 [46], urged member countries to use the resources of traditional medicine and complementary, that will be investigated so that these resources enjoy efficacy and safety and that they are incorporated into the national health system, making a follow-up for its evaluation.

2.4 The challenges in health in the twenty-first century

High infant mortality in developing countries continues to be the great scourge worldwide, in contrast to the increase in life expectancy in developed countries [47]. The unequal distribution of wealth has a negative impact on education, and the lack of it is the gateway to all kinds of ills. Economic poverty is associated with crime, unemployment, precarious housing and increased morbidity. On the contrary, countries with a higher economic level, with a national public health system, private or mixed, with the predominant medical paradigm, experience an increase in life expectancy, with an increase in chronic diseases that, with they often reduce the quality of life and entail high human and material costs, seriously endangering their economic sustainability [48].

The Lalonde report on the health determinants of 1974 made it clear that what influences our state of health the most is the lifestyle we adopt and, what is less, health care, however, the greatest expense fell on the latter [49]. In 1978, the meeting of health experts from Alma-Ata in Kazakhstan (which belonged at that time to the former Soviet Union), established Primary Health Care as the ideal framework for prevention and health promotion [50]. In successive international conferences on health (see **Table 1**) it has been tried to carry out these purposes, until arriving at the Astana meeting in 2018, which took stock of these 40 years.

In September 2000, the leaders of the world met at the United Nations Headquarters in New York and adopted the Millennium Declaration, committing their countries to a new global alliance to reduce the levels of extreme poverty and establishing a series of objectives with goals and indicators, known as the Millennium Development Goals (MDGs) until the 2015 period. The MDGs sought developing countries to take new measures and join efforts in the fight against poverty, illiteracy, hunger, lack of education, gender inequality, infant and maternal mortality, HIV infection and environmental degradation. Other objectives called for developed countries to adopt measures to relieve debt, increase assistance to developing countries and promote a fairer market [51]. In 2015, the States agreed on a new agenda for development, that of 2030 [52].

The 2030 Development Agenda is a plan of action in favor of people, the planet and prosperity. It also aims to strengthen universal peace within a broader concept of freedom. The adoption of the SDGs represented a historic opportunity to unite countries and people from all over the world and to take new paths to the future. The SDGs are formulated to eradicate poverty, promote prosperity and well-being for all, protect the environment and tackle global climate change. The Astana meeting in Kazakhstan (formerly Alma-Ata) of 2018 had objectives to reinforce Primary Health Care (PHC), achieve universal health coverage and sustainable development objectives. In his point V he stressed that we had to work to make PHC sustainable. As in the Shanghai conference, it was insisted on empowering people and the community in its VI point.

Thus, the prevention of diseases and the promotion of health, is to rewrite the functions of PHC (health centers), currently focused on the resolution of problems with the use of drugs, causing iatrogenic and high health expenditure, jeopardizing its economic sustainability [53]. It is necessary to reshape the PHC focusing on the individualization, the transmission of positive information, the modification of unhealthy behavior, the medical advice, all within a procedure of humanization of health care, something deteriorated since the arrival of technology and the economic crisis.

Conference	Date	Theme/objectives/performances
Ottawa	1986	The promotion of health in the general context of globalization
Adelaide	1988	Formulation of healthy policies
Sundsvall	1991	Creating enabling environments
Yakarta	1997	Capacity building for health promotion
México	2000	Capacity building for health promotion
Bangkok	2005	The promotion of health in the general context of globalization
Nairobi	2009	Actions to reduce the gap between the evidence and its concrete application in the development of health
Helsinki	2013	Health in all policies
Shanghai	2016	Declaration of Shanghai (2030 agenda for sustainable development)
Astaná	2018	Review of the 40 years of Alma-Ata

Compiled by A. Ursa. WHO Global Health Promotion Conferences.

Table 1.
International conferences on health promotion.

2.5 Medicine and climate change

The Intergovernmental Panel on Climate Change (IPCC) was created in 1988 by the World Meteorological Organization (WMO) and the United Nations (UN) in its United Nations Environment Program (UNEP), with the objective of providing an objective source of scientific information. The main activity of the IPCC is to publish special reports on issues relevant to the implementation of the United Nations Framework Convention on Climate Change (UNFCCC). The IPCC has published five comprehensive reports examining the latest climate evidence, as well as numerous special reports on particular issues.

In 1997, the Kyoto Protocol on climate change was drafted with the objective of reducing emissions of the main greenhouse gases such as carbon dioxide, methane, nitrous oxide, sulfur hexafluoride, hydrofluorocarbons and perfluorocarbons [54]. The successive meetings of climate change experts and some of their conclusions appear in **Table 2**.

Throughout these years there has been a slow progress on compliance with the agreements on the reduction of greenhouse gases. The most industrialized countries put obstacles to their accession, placing their own interests before the generals. Objective 13 of the 2030 Agenda for Sustainable Development requires urgent actions to combat climate change and its impacts and is intrinsically related to the other 16 objectives of the Agenda.

Although global warming may have some beneficial effects, such as lower winter mortality in temperate regions and an increase in food production in certain areas, the overall health effects are likely to be very damaging [54]. Climate change influences the social and environmental determinants of health, such as clean air, clean water, sufficient food and safe housing. The countries that have contributed least to greenhouse gas emissions will be the first and most affected by climate change [55].

The emergence of extreme downpours with floods, alternating with droughts is likely to cause famine and increase morbidity and mortality in countries with fewer

Meetings	Date	Agreements
Río de Janeiro	1992	Creation of the UNFCCC
Kyoto (Japan)	1997	Kyoto Protocol with binding legal objectives
Balí (Indonesia)	2007	Road map of Bali (post-Kyoto)
Copenhague	2009	Agreement de Copenhague
Cancún	2010	Reactivation of the greenhouse gas reduction pact del
Durban	2011	Commitment to extend the Kyoto Protocol
Doha (Qatar)	2012	2020 climate change agreement
Varsovia	2013	Warsaw International Mechanism
Perú	2014	Commitment to seal the Paris Agreement
París	2015	Paris Agreement
Marrakech	2016	Declaration of support for the Paris Agreement
Bonn	2017	Its objective is to accelerate the fulfillment of the objectives of the Paris Agreement
Katowice	2018	Katowice book
Madrid	2019	Agreement, called "Chile-Madrid to Act"

Compiled by A. Ursa of the author Vengoechea, of the Friedrich Ebert Foundation, 2012.

Table 2.
Meetings on climate change/summits of the earth.

resources [56]. There will be an important transfer of climate refugees between countries that may trigger conflicts of various kinds. Heat waves will cause more deaths, especially at extreme ages. Climate change could alter the geographical distribution of disease vectors, such as insects that transmit malaria or dengue [57]. It is expected that, between 2030 and 2050, climate change will cause an additional 250,000 deaths each year, due to malnutrition, malaria, diarrhea and heat stress. It is estimated that the cost of direct damage to health (that is, excluding costs in the determinant sectors for health, such as agriculture and water and sanitation) is between 2000 and 4000 million US dollars from here 2030 [58].

2.6 The change of model as a solution to climate change

For more than 200 years, the temperature of the Earth has been going upward due to human activity. The Earth ecosystem is sensitive to this progressive rise in temperature and is experiencing damaging effects on seas, the mainland and the atmosphere. The consequences that we face are already felt. The international bodies meet to seek solutions for years, but they are insufficient and the most powerful countries, which pollute the most, do not adopt the resolutions so that, supposedly, they do not influence their economy.

As international consensus measures, the change in the energy model is presented, with the progressive abandonment of fossil fuel burning and replacement with renewable energies. The proposed deadlines are not very ambitious and the implementation times will have to be shortened, because the forecasts fall short again and again. The feeding model established in the last decades based on animal protein results in poorer health, with an increase in type 2 diabetes mellitus and cardiovascular diseases [59].

The cattle and sheep farming, through the emission of methane in its digestive process, contributes a good amount to climate change. The other major emitter is transport by land, sea and air. A scarce resource is water. One kilogram of beef consumes approximately 20,000 L of water. It is deforested in ancestral forests to plant soy and corn, to produce feed for cattle [60].

However, meat consumption is increasing worldwide, especially in emerging countries (China, North Africa, etc.). Experts advise to modify the diet to be healthier and reduce the environmental impact, reducing the consumption of meat and increasing the legumes, vegetables and fruits [61]. Returning to the Alma-Ata model and ratified in Astana in 2018, primary health care must insist on the prevention and promotion of health, empowering the user, advising the adoption of a healthy lifestyle and raising awareness of the impact that they have our actions in climate change [62].

For broader coverage of the health system, international organizations should make proposals to the most disadvantaged countries to adopt cheap and proven public health interventions to control climate-sensitive diseases, in line with the achievement of the Goals of Millennium development related to health (currently sustainable development goals) [63]. Climate change is a price we are paying for misguided global policies. The achievement of economic wealth prevailed over the protection of the health of the planet and of the most vulnerable sectors of society. We must insist on the implementation of the resolutions adopted by international organizations in order to reduce the global impact of climate change.

3. Conclusions

The pillars of well-being that have been achieved in many western countries can be threatened by different scenarios, such as climate change, armed conflicts,

DOI: http://dx.doi.org/10.5772/intechopen.88384

trade wars, population aging or migratory flows caused by the above circumstances. The solutions to these problems include the adoption of international agreements that reduce greenhouse gas emissions, accelerate the energy transition with the use of renewable energy, reduce meat consumption, improve health promotion at the first level (primary health care) and the distribution of the resources offered by the Earth is improved, with a more sustainable management. Following the recommendations of the World Health Organization, alternative and complementary medicines should be promoted and resources allocated to research to those who enjoy scientific evidence, in order to cover greater coverage of the population both in Western countries and in those countries with a poor health system, without giving up the current scientific-technical medicine.

Abbreviations

IPCC	Intergovernmental Panel on Climate Change
MDG	Millennium Development Goals (Millennium Declaration)
SDG	Sustainable development goals
UN	Organization of the United Nations
UNEP	United Nations Environment Program
UNFCCC	United Nations Framework Convention on Climate Change
WHO	World Health Organization
WMO	World Meteorological Organization
PHC	Primary health care

Author details

Andrés J. Ursa Herguedas[1,2,3]

1 Junta de Castilla y León, Spain

2 Illustrious Academy of Health Sciences Ramón y Cajal, Madrid, Spain

3 Institute of Integrative Medicine, Valladolid, Spain

*Address all correspondence to: ajursa@educa.jcyl.es

References

[1] Carasa P. For a social history of the city. Urbanization, pauperism and assistance. In: Bonamusa F, Serrallonga J, editors. The Urban Society. Barcelona: Association of Contemporary History; 1994. pp. 23-55

[2] Hans-Martin F, et al. Climate Change, Impacts and Vulnerability in Europe 2016. Vol. 1. Luxembourg: European Environment Agency; 2017. DOI: 10.2800/534806

[3] Latest review of science reveals ocean in critical state from cumulative impacts. In: Rogers A, Laffoley D, editors. International Programme on the State of the Ocean. London; 2013. Available from: http://www.sciencedirect.com/science/journal/0025326X/74

[4] Ferlay J et al. Cancer Incidence and Mortality Worldwide. Vol. 11. Lyon, France: International Center for Cancer Research; 2013. DOI: 10.1002/ijc.29210

[5] Laín Entralgo P. Hippocratic Medicine. 1st ed. Madrid: University Alliance; 1982. p. 19. Available from: http://www.cervantesvirtual.com/nd/ark:/59851/bmc99027

[6] Laín Entralgo P. History of Medicine. Reprint. Salvat Editores. Barcelona: S.A.; 1978. p. 17. Available from: http://www.cervantesvirtual.com/nd/ark:/59851/bmcqj991

[7] Álvarez SE. Acupuncture Treatise. PAR. Madrid: Graphic Arts S.A.; 1983. p. 33. ISBN-13: 978-8430089031

[8] Caldecott T. Ayurveda: The Divine Science of Life. Edimburg U.K.: Elsevier Health Sciences; 2006. ISBN: 9780723434108

[9] Stone Potter D, Mattingly DJ. Life, Death and Entertainment in the Roman Empire. In: Potters DS, Mattingley DJ, editors. Ann Arbor EEUU, USA: University of Michigan Press; 1999. p. 63. ISBN: 0-472-08568-9

[10] Abü Bakr Muhammad ibn Zakariya al Razi. The Book of Spiritual Medicine. Translation of Tornero. In: Trotta, editor. Trotta Police. Leaflets from the East. Madrid; 2004

[11] Gutas D. Avicenna and the Aristotelian Tradition: Introduction to Reading Avicenna's Philosophical Works. Leiden: Brill; 1988. DOI: 10.15808/Nazariyat.1.2.D0016

[12] Hernández MC, ibn Rushd (Averroes) A-l-W M. Life, Work, Thought, Influence. 2nd ed. Córdoba: Caja Sur Publications; 1997. ISSN 1136-8071

[13] Aguinis M. Maimónides. Buenos Aires: Jewish People's Library; 1976

[14] Capparoni P. Magistri Salernitani Nondum Cogniti. A Contribution to the History of the Medical School of Salerno. Londres: Bale& Danielsson; 1923

[15] González PA. Don Ramón and the Translators of Toledo. In: Labor, editor. Madrid; 1942

[16] Paniagua Arellano JA. Studies and notes on Arnau de Vilanova. Madrid: Superior Council of Scientific Investigations (CSIC); 1963

[17] Borelli BG. Life Series of Famous Doctors and Naturalists. Trieste; 1947

[18] Riviere P. Paracelso. Barcelona: Ed De Vecchi; 2001. ISBN: 978-84-315-2642-9

[19] Kushner H., Cortes D.: Sydenham's chorea. In: Koehler Peter J. u_a (Hrsg): Neurological Eponyms. Oxford: Oxford University Press; 2000. ISBN: 0-19-513366-8

[20] Coulston Gillispie C, Lawrence HF, Koertge N. In: Gale T, editor. Complete Dictionary of Scientific Biography. Detroit, Michigan: Charles Scribner's Sons; 2008. ISBN: 9780684315591 0684315599

[21] Demangeon JB. Historical Painting of a Triple Establishment Gathered in a Single Hospice in Copenhagen. Paris; año VII. 1871

[22] Grandjean de Fouchy JP. In praise of M. Morgagni. In: History of the Royal Academy of Sciences. Vol. 1774. Paris: Imprimerie Royale; 1771. pp. 131-142

[23] Hahnemann S. The Organon of the Healing Art. 6th ed. Barcelona, Spain: Homeopathic Institute of Catalonia; 2012. ISBN: 9788461569229

[24] Berriot-Salvadore E. The discourse of medicine and science. In: History of Women. Vol. 3. From the Renaissance to the Modern Age. Buenos Aires: Santillana, S.A., Taurus minor; 1993. pp. 385-431

[25] Burci C. Summarized History of Italian Surgery from its Beginning until the Nineteenth Century. Florencia; 1876. pp. 43-44

[26] Figueiredo BG. Bleeders and surgeons: Medical practitioners in nineteenth century Minas Gerais. History, Sciences, Health-Manguinhos. 1999;**6**(2):277-291. DOI: 10.1590/S0104-59701999000300003

[27] Salas-Salvado J et al. Food and Nutrition throughout History. Glosa Ed. Barcelona, Spain; 2005

[28] Rodríguez PH. Medical Hydrology Manual. Barcelona (Spain): Reus Eds; 1925

[29] Cannon WB. The Wisdom of the Body. New York: Norton & Company, Inc.; 1932

[30] Bloch H. Edward Jenner (1749-1823). The history and effects of smallpox, inoculation, and vaccination. American Journal of Diseases of Children. 1993;**147**(7):772-774. ISSN: 0002-922X

[31] Collard P. The Development of Microbiology. UK: Cambridge University Press; 1976

[32] Schmalstieg FC Jr, Goldman AS. Ilya Ilich Metchnikoff (1845-1915) and Paul Ehrlich (1854-1915): The centennial of the 1908 Nobel prize in physiology or medicine. Journal of Medical Biography. 2008;**16**(2):96-103. DOI: 10.1258/jmb.2008.008006

[33] Cordón F. History of Biochemistry. Madrid (Spain): Compañía literaria S.L.; 1997

[34] Glasser O. Wilhelm Conrad Röntgen and the Early History of the Roentgen Rays. Londres (UK): John Bale, Sons and Danielsson Ltd.; 1933. ISBN: 0930405226

[35] Bringmann U. The foundation of the Institute of Experimental Psychology at the University of Leipzig. Psychological Research. 1990;**42**:13

[36] Planck M. Scientific Autobiography and Latest Writings. In: Nivola, editor. New York, USA; 2000. ISBN: 9780806530758

[37] Dunn LC. A Short History of Genetics. Nueva York: McGraw-Hill; 1965

[38] Virchow RLK. Cellular Pathology. 1859 special ed. London, UK: John Churchill; 1978

[39] Font QP. Medicinal Plants. The Dioscorides Renewed. 5th ed. Barcelona: Labor S.A.; 1979

[40] Vélez LP. On the notion, meaning and importance of the Toledo school. Disputatio Philosophical Research Bulletin. 2017;**6**(7):537-579

[41] Conrad L, Nutton V, et al. The Western Medical Traditions: 800 BC to AD 1800. Cambridge, UK: Cambridge University Press; 1995

[42] Leclerc H. Precise Phytotherapy: Therapeutic Trial by French Plants. Paris, France: Masson; 1983. Paperback

[43] Mulet Salort JM. Natural Products, What a Scam! Pamplona (Navarra) Spain: Laetoli; 2011. ISBN: 9788492422289

[44] Rakel D. Integrative Medicine. 2nd ed. Barcelona: Elsevier Masson; 2009. p. 7. ISBN: 987-84-458-1911-1

[45] Resolution WHA 62.13. Traditional Medicine; 2009

[46] Resolution WHA 67.18. Traditional Medicine; 2014

[47] Dhrifi A. Expenses in health, economic growth and infant mortality: History of developed and developing countries. CEPAL Review. 2018;**125**:69-91

[48] Foreman K et al. Prognosis of life expectancy, years of life lost and mortality from all causes and specific causes for 250 causes of death: Reference and alternative scenarios for 2016-40 for 195 countries and territories using data from the global study of burden of diseases. The Lancet. 2018;**392**:2052-2090. DOI: 10.1016/S0140-6736(18)31694-5

[49] Lalonde M. A New Perspectives on the Health of Canadians. Ottawa, Canadá: Government of Canada; 1974. Available from: http://www.phac-aspc.gc.ca/ph-sp/pdf/perspect-eng.pdf

[50] International Conference on Primary Health Care. Alma-Ata: World Health Organization (WHO), UNICEFF; 1978. ISBN: 92 4 354135 8

[51] United Nations Millennium Declaration, 55/2. New York; 2000. Available from: http://undocs.org/A/RES/55/2

[52] United Nations. Sustainable Development Objectives. New York: United Nations, General Assembly; 2015. Available from: https://onu.org.gt/objetivos-de-desarrollo/

[53] Gervás J et al. (SESPAS report 2012). Health expenditure on primary care in Spain: Not enough to provide attractive services to patients and health professionals. Medical Gazette. 2012;**26**(S1):36-40

[54] Kyoto Protocol, United Nations Framework Convention on Climate Change. New York: UN; 1998

[55] Intergovernmental Panel on Climate Change (IPCC). Summary for policy makers. In: Edenhofer O, Pichs-Madruga R, Sokona Y, Farahani E, Kadner S, Seyboth K, Adler A, et al. editors. Climate Change 2014: Mitigation of Climate Change. Contribution of Working Group III to the Fifth Assessment Report of the IPCC. Cambridge, United Kingdom and New York, NY, USA: Cambridge University Press; 2014. UU. Chapter 11. ISBN: 978-1-107-05821-7

[56] McMichael A, Campbell-Lendrum D, Kovats R, et al. Climate change. In: Ezzati M, Lopez A, Rodgers A, Murray C, dir. Publ. Comparative Quantification of Health Risks: Global and Regional Burden of Disease Due to Selected Major Risk Factors. WHO (Ginebra). 2004. DOI: doi:10.1016/S0140-6736(09)61993-0

[57] Ebi KL, Boven K. Extreme events as sources of health vulnerability: Drought as an example. Weather and Climate Extremes. 2016;**11**:95-102. ISBN: 978-1-107-02506-6

[58] WHO. Special Report COP24: Health and Climate Change.

Geneva, Switzerland; 2018. ISBN: 978-92-4-151497-2

[59] Micha R et al. Red and processed meat consumption and risk of incident coronary heart disease, stroke and diabetes mellitus: A systematic review and metaanalysis. The Circulation. 2010;**121**(21):2271-2283. DOI: 10.1161/CIRCULATIONAHA.109.924977

[60] Steinfeld H, Gerber P, Wassenaar T, Castel V, Rosales M, de Haan C. Livestick's Long Shadow. Environmental Issues and Options. Roma: FAO; 2006. ISBN: 978-92-5-105571-7

[61] Rose D, Heller MC, Roberto CA. Position of the Society for Education and Nutritional Behavior: The importance of including environmental sustainability in dietary guidance. Journal of Nutrition Education and Behavior. 2019;**51**(1):3-15. DOI: 10.1016/j.jneb.2018.07.006

[62] Declaration of Astana. In: Global Conference on Primary Health Care; 25 and 26 October, 2018; Astana (Kazakhstan). 2018. Available from: https://bit.ly/2Rm8TTv

[63] Millennium Declaration 55/2. New York: UN; 2000

Chapter 7

Seasonal Changes of Soil Organic Carbon and Microbial Biomass Carbon in Different Forest Ecosystems

Emre Babur and Turgay Dindaroglu

Abstract

Soil organic carbon (SOC) and microbial biomass carbon (MBC) are important components of soil organic matter (SOM). SOC and MBC have generally recognized key parameters of soil quality and health, and also they have been linked to forest ecosystem productivity, using as a sensitive indicator for ecosystem monitoring programs. Both of them play a crucial role in the carbon cycle and influence many environmental, biological, and chemical factors. Soil organic matter decomposition by soil microorganisms contributes to the nutrient availability and release in an ecosystem. This interaction between SOM and MBC is managed in soil aggregation, soil porosity, moisture content, and aeration. Forest soils can store more carbon than other land uses because they contain a wide variety of soil microorganisms. Enhancing these two important components of soil can contribute to climate change mitigation and adaptation strategies. In this chapter, an overview of the understanding of the most important soil quality and health factors managed soil C in forest soils and provided how seasonal changes affect soil organic carbon and microbial biomass carbon.

Keywords: forest soils, seasonal change, soil organic carbon, microbial biomass, soil health

1. Introduction

Soil is one of the most important components of ecosystems. It provides plant growth by regulating the cycling of nutrients, energy, and water. Also, soils play a major role in the carbon cycle among the atmosphere, vegetation, land, and ocean. Soil organic carbon (SOC) stores approximately 1600 PgC in the 100 cm depth, which contains more carbon than in the terrestrial vegetation (approx. 600 PgC) and in the atmosphere (approx. 800 PgC) [1, 2]. The carbon cycle is the exchanges between the various carbon reservoirs: biosphere, lithosphere, atmosphere, ocean, and fossil fuels (**Figure 1**).

In the last decades, atmospheric C concentration is known to increase with anthropogenic carbon emissions (ACEs) (e.g. fossil fuel combustion and cement manufacturing). The ACE was 6 Pg year^{-1} in the 1980s [3]; it had increased to 10 Pg year^{-1} in 2014 [4]. This caused a significant increase in global warming (**Figure 2**).

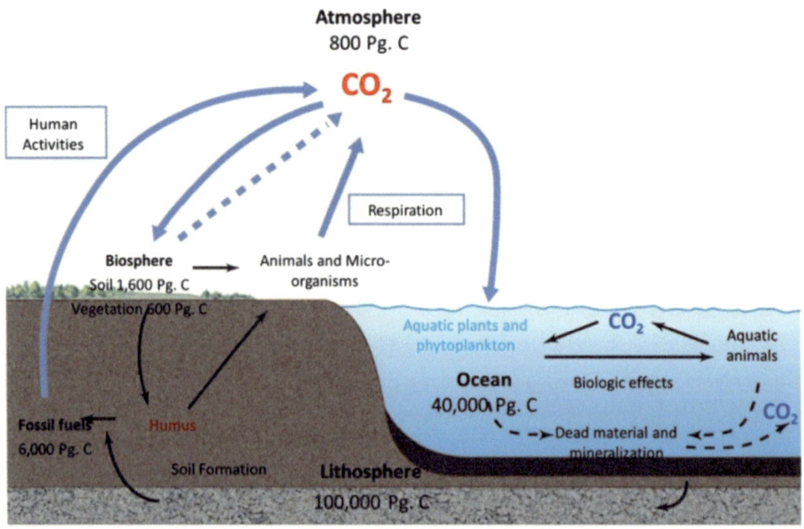

Figure 1.
The global carbon cycle and carbon reservoirs.

Forest ecosystems contain terrestrial C since they store huge quantities of carbon in different pools such as vegetation, litter, and soil and exchange big amounts of C with the atmosphere through respiration and photosynthesis. Among the OC reservoirs in forests, the soil stores *large quantities* of OC, accumulating C as soil organic matter (SOM). Indeed, soils have been accepted as the largest terrestrial carbon pool because of the greater C content than terrestrial vegetation and atmospheric C [5, 6]. Forest soil can friendly contribute to reducing the atmospheric carbon dioxide concentration and the greenhouse effect in global warming, while the soil is considered a big carbon pool [7, 8], linked to the carbon cycle [5] and with the nutrient pool that assigns vegetation productivity [9].

In recent years, the researchers have focused on the SOM properties and soil organic carbon (SOC) which can have significant effects on its dynamics and also the direction of ecosystem reactions related to climate change (e.g., decomposition time, increasing soil temperature and CO_2 levels or changes in composition of vegetation, N deposition, etc.) [11, 12]. Most studies of SOC are related to soil fertility, soil management, SOM decomposition, and effects of greenhouse gas emissions in climate change. SOM is a significantly important factor in soil quality and productivity; however, this alone does not help adequately predict any changes in soil quality and nutrient status [13, 14].

The SOM decomposition process is dependent on substrate type and quality (fragment type and size, decay stage, nutrient availability, and tree species) and amount and activity of the soil microorganisms and environmental factors (climate, soil texture, structure, soil chemical compounds, soil moisture and temperature, aggregation soil nutrient availability and temperature, etc.) [15–20]. For example, though the soils under tropical forests store the highest amount of OC, desert soil stores the lowest amount of OC [21, 22]. Soil silt and clay content maintains organic carbon by aggregation [15, 23]. Hassink [19] revealed an increase in the SOC stored in the <20 μm size fraction with an increase of clay + silt content. The soil sample has been shown under a microscope in **Figure 3**. Moreover, Gabarron-Galeote et al. [24] found that the highest soil carbon content is found in the silt and clay size fractions than the sand fractions.

Especially, studies on soil C dynamics and its effect on the global carbon cycle have been increased: (1) the importance of SOC for microbial biomass carbon (MBC) in dimension beyond a depth of 20 cm [17, 20, 25]; (2) the interaction

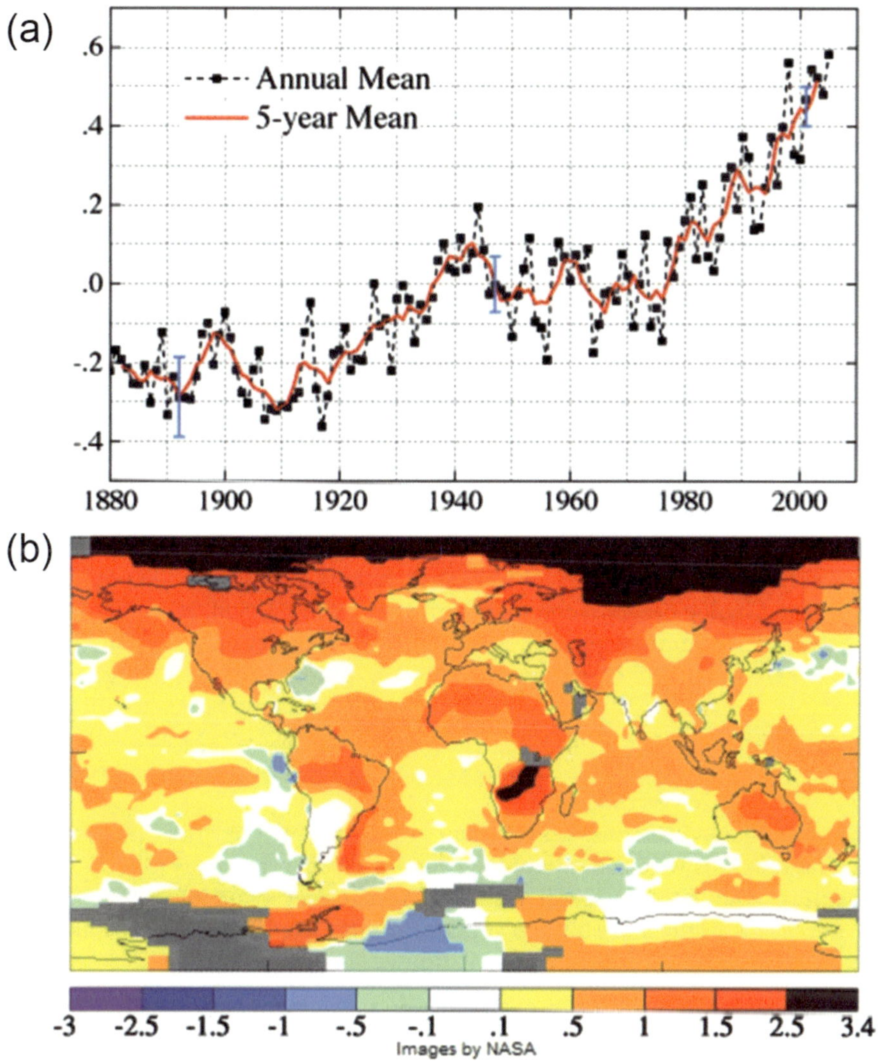

Figure 2.
Annual temperature increase (a) and degree of increase (b) in worldwide. Source: images by NASA [10].

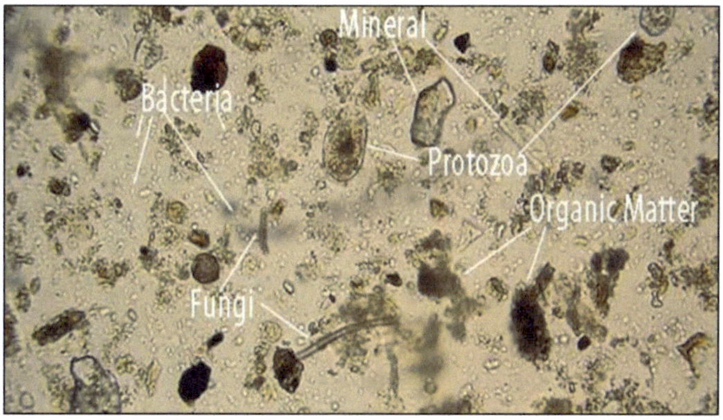

Figure 3.
Soil sample under microscope by mauby.com [28].

between microbial communities and its activity with soil properties in relation to the carbon cycle and with other nutrient cycles [26, 27]; and (3) the effects of plant species in increasing soil microbial biomass and soil carbon storage [17].

2. Soil organic carbon in forest ecosystem

Forest ecosystems have been long accepted the most efficient tools for carbon sinks that can reduce atmospheric emissions via carbon sequestration in soil and plant biomass and directly reduce greenhouse effect [29]. Forest soils containing more than 70% of all the soil organic carbon are sequestered by forest ecosystems [30]. Therefore, in the use of forest soils against global climate change, the processes of organic matter cycle in soil and the site factors governing these processes need to be carefully evaluated. In other words we need to know the characteristics and interaction among ecosystems, plants, and soil in forests [31]. In forest ecosystems, SOM can be used as a significant indicator of soil quality and site productivity [32]. Since soil organic matter is composed of the higher amount of dead plant mass (forest floor and dead wood) and animals, OM is higher in forests than other land-use types. Also, the productivity of forest ecosystems depends on soil physical, chemical, and biological characteristics and processes [31]. Soil OC is one of the most essential soil components that contributes to ecosystem productivity through its positive effects on soil structure, aeration, and porosity and maintaining soil water and temperature [33–35]. Moreover, SOM has a strong relation with nutrient availability, because it is an important nutrient source that can be used by plants in long periods. Besides, SOM contributes to forming soil structure and increases water holding capacity in soils.

In recent years, numerous studies have been conducted to state the carbon stocks and relations with soil microbial communities in forest soils [30, 36–42], and other studies conducted on seasonal changes in soil microbial biomass [20, 43–47]. On the other hand, there are limited studies for more sequestering atmospheric C in soils by increasing microorganism populations.

3. Soil microbial biomass carbon in forest ecosystem

The terrestrial carbon cycle is provided by photosynthesis and respiratory balance. Carbon fixation by autotrophs, photosynthetic plants, and photo-chemotrophic microorganisms allows the transfer of carbon from the atmosphere to the soil. The return of carbon to the atmosphere takes place through the fossil fuels and respiration of microbial and other organisms. Soil microorganisms utilize carbon sources around the main objectives for growth and proliferation. Therefore, microbes use different forms of organic and inorganic carbon as carbon and energy sources. Due to the role of microorganism activities in the carbon cycle, it interacts directly and indirectly with climate change. For example, organic C mineralization and CO_2 released by respiration increase with increasing temperature. The amount of CO_2 accumulated in the soil increases photosynthesis and release of root exudates. This leads to microbial decomposition and respiratory instability. Since soil microorganisms in the carbon cycle have an important role, soil microbial biomass is utilized in most carbon cycle models. Soil microbial activity rate indicates the potential and dynamics of the nutrient cycle in a particular ecosystem. Also, microbial properties of soils can be used as an indicator of any fluctuations in the ecosystem due to its sensitivity to weather conditions, plant species or in the characteristics of animal residues [36, 48]. Soil microbial respiration is one of the most important microbial indices first calculated in the majority of models. Microbial soil respiration explains all activity or energy consumption of the microbial communities [49]; therefore, it is the main parameter to observe decomposition rate [50].

The soil microorganisms are small, containing about 2–3% of SOC. But they are very important component in ecosystem function basically through the regulation carbon sequestering, soil respiration, plant productivity and also related to the nutrient mineralization, which plays a crucial role in the biogeochemical cycling of carbon (C), nitrogen (N), and phosphorus (P) in continental ecosystems [36, 37, 51–53]. SMB is the dynamic fraction of soil organic matter, which includes fungi, bacteria, actinomycetes, algae, protozoa, and other microfauna (**Figure 4**) and demonstrates an important nutrient pool in the soil [37]. Soil nutrient conservation processes and transformation are greatly interrelated to the amount of microbial biomass present in the soil (**Figure 5**).

Soil microorganisms are the active agent of soil organic matter and the most dynamic factor in soil. Hence, soil microbiological or biochemical characteristics are much more susceptible to any changes in soil conditions (degradation, erosion) and supply more accurate and immediate information in soil health and quality [54, 55]. For example, any changes in microbial biomass can be detected rapidly and precisely when compared to changes in soil physicochemical properties [56–58]. Nowadays, international programs for monitoring soil health and quality department noticed that combining the measurement of several microbial indices such as soil microbial diversity, microbial biomass, microbial respiration, and soil enzymes should be determined to measure ecosystem health [40, 50, 59] (**Table 1**). Insam et al. [60] also recommended that the ratio of microbial biomass to total organic carbon might state as an indicator of carbon dynamics in the soil. For example, microorganisms are extremely influenced by anthropogenic effects such as irrigation, fertilization, using insecticide, conventional tillage, etc. [61, 62]. The importance of microorganisms in ecosystem functioning has caused to proliferate the interest in determining soil microbial properties [63]. Soil microbial biomass is a source of microbial biomass carbon (MBC), microbial biomass nitrogen (MBN), microbial biomass phosphorus (MBP), and microbial biomass sulfur (MBS).

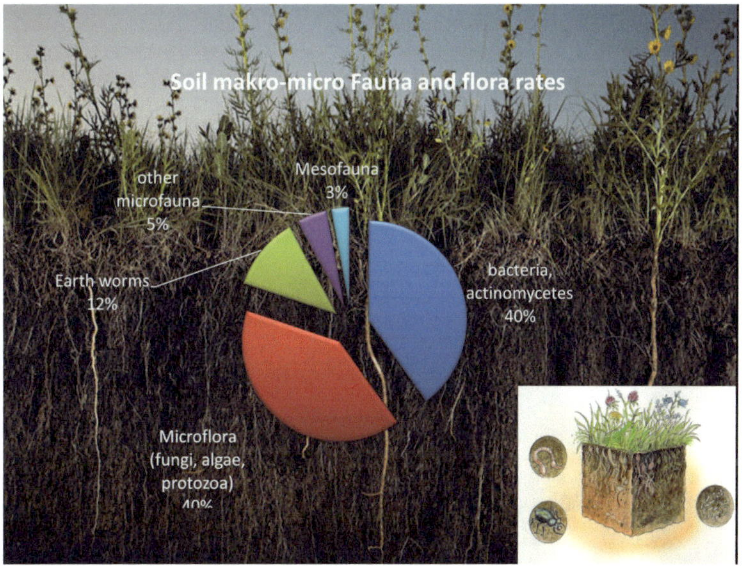

Figure 4.
Soil macro-micro fauna and flora rates.

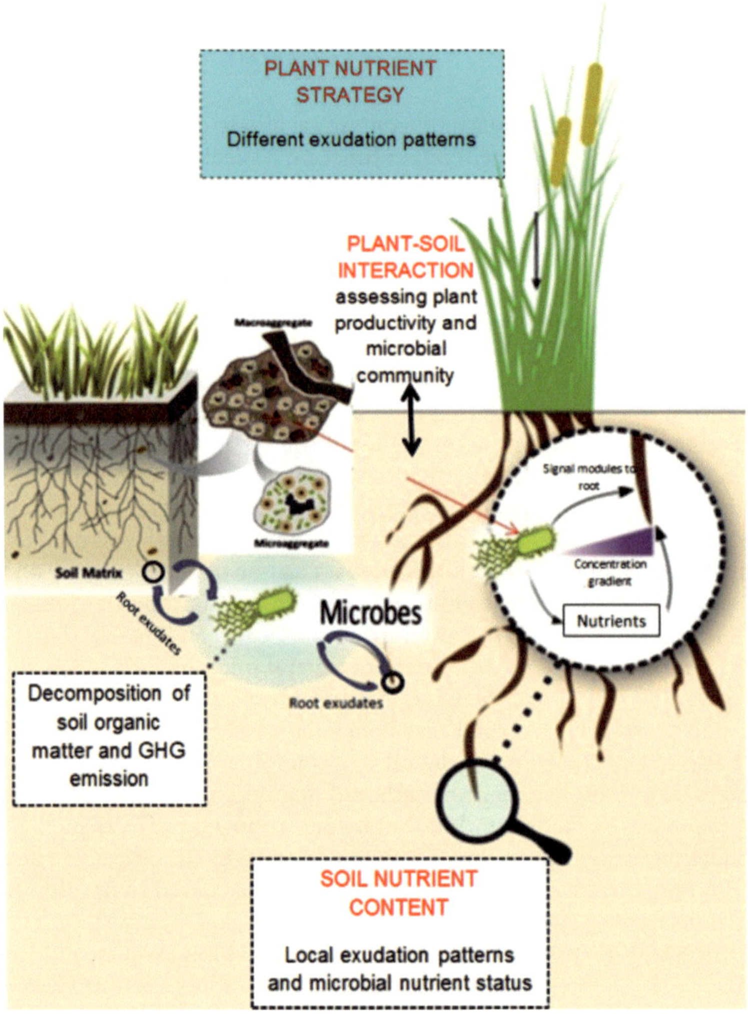

Figure 5.
The figure illustrates a summary of the concepts proposed for the role of root exudates in plantmicrobe interactions and consequences for ecosystems. Source: By changing from Canarini et al. [65].

Properties	• Soil mineralogy	• pH	• Microbial biomass
	• Texture	• Electrical conductivity	• Basal respiration
	• Soil depth	• Cation-exchange capacity	• N mineralization
	• Bulk density	• Organic matter	• Enzyme activities
	• Water holding capacity	• Macro-nutrition elements	• Micro-flora community
	• Porosity	• Heavy metals	• Plant biodiversity
			• Root diseases
			• Plant growth

Table 1.
Physical, chemical and biological soil properties used as indicators in determining soil quality (changed from Pankhurst et al. [58]).

The MBC and MBN comprise 1–5% and 2–6% of the total soil C and N contents and tend to be relatively more stable. Approximately 1.4% of the world's soil organic C content comprises soil MBC, but it contributes significantly to the global C cycle [64].

Soil microbial biomass plays a significant role in linking the plants and soil. A variety of plant species can influence soil characteristics, soil microbial composition and activity via their root activity, the release of root exudates, exogenous enzymes, sloughed-off cells, lysates, and litter decomposition into the rhizosphere [17, 66–68]. Exudates of plant halophytic roots supply sources of energy and carbon to microbes, considering that vegetation type, vegetation growth stage, metabolism type, and seasonal change are the main factors that influence the root exudates quantity and quality [69–71]. Thanks to different growth patterns, root structure and development, and resource distribution of different plants can lead to different microbial communities and their activity [69]. Richards et al. [72] and Malchair et al. [73] found that changes in tree species and composition potentially affect SOM quantity and dynamics. Additionally, some environmental factors such as moisture, temperature, and seasons influence soil microbial activities and result in changes in key biogeochemical cycles [71, 74]. The decomposition of SOM begins with enzyme-mediated hydrolysis of complex substrates, and these enzyme activities are used as indicators of soil quality [67, 75]. Bolat et al. [76] found that black locust trees significantly affect the total nitrogen (TN) content of the soil, because of the enzymatic activity and N-fixing ability by roots. It is also noticed that the SOC and TN content occurs due to the decomposition and accumulation of organic material in soils [77–79]. If organic material is added to a soil, it is decomposed by soil microorganisms and converted into some nutrients such as C, N, P, and K which are released in the soil.

Among the soil microbial indices, the soil microbial respiration is influenced by seasonal patterns, but seasonal change directly influences soil metabolism or indirectly affects the changes in microbial community composition and substrate availability. Determining any changes in microbial biomass C and N contents is important in a terrestrial ecosystem. However, many previous studies reveal that it is difficult to determine how changes in soil microbial biomass are regulated [80, 81].

Numerous studies have been conducted on the soil microbial biomass in different forest ecosystems [38–40, 82, 83], and also other studies that focused on seasonal changes in soil microbial biomass [43–45, 47, 84–88]. In general, some soil properties differ in the year. Zhou et al. [89] found that the changes in soil biomass in tropical and subtropical regions are higher in the summer than in the winter. This study noticed that whether moisture and temperature directly influence the soil community and biochemical processes.

Seasonal changes affect the soil temperature, soil moisture, organic matter content, root activity and amount of microbial community, and composition causing fluctuations in the soil. Also, these changes vary according to soil texture, structure, vegetation diversity and type, land-use type, and management application [87, 90]. Investigating the seasonal changes of microbial activities and biomass is essential for a better understanding of the nutrient dynamics in tree plantation.

4. Relationship between soil microbial biomass and organic carbon

Soil quality and health indicate the condition of the soil, depending on the chemical, physical, and biological factors that manage the biogeochemical processes of the soil. Some soil properties are rapidly affected by changes in environmental factors; other soil properties, which are not suitable for assessing soil health and quality, change very slowly in a long time [78, 91–92]. For instance, some studies have noticed that soil microbial indexes and activity may use more rapid indicators of soil health and quality than the physical and chemical soil properties (e.g., OC and TN). Therefore, soil's biochemical characteristics (e.g., MBC, MBN, C_{mic}/C_{org}

percentage, C_{mic}/N_{mic} ratio, basal respiration, and qCO_2 ratio) respond immediately to environmental stress [50, 57, 93].

Soils that have a high OC content usually have higher microbial biomass quantities [20, 39, 76, 94]. SOM decomposition by soil microorganisms plays a crucial role in global carbon and nitrogen cycling [95]. Substrate quality (e.g., lignin, cellulose, hemicellulose content) and the labile C and nutrient availability significantly affect soil microbial decomposition [96, 97]. The availability of nutrient sources affects the decomposition processes by influencing microbial physiology such as the production of extracellular enzyme activities. When there is an insufficient available nutrient or substrate, the microbial production of extracellular enzymes is stimulated [98–100]. Winding et al. [101] noticed that soil biogeochemical process can be determined by organic matter degradation or basal respiration, and it provides an estimation of microbial activity rate. A variety of microbial activities may show differences in the organic carbon cycle and nutrients within the terrestrial ecosystem. Also, Insam et al. [102] reported that the metabolic quotient (qCO2) can be an indicator of soil development and decreases with ecological succession. For the abovementioned reasons, it is necessary to know the microbial properties of the soil for nutrient cycle balance and soil quality indicating plant growth.

5. Seasonal changes of SOC and SMBC

Seasonal changes have a significant effect on the soil OC, microbial biomass C and N, and other related microbial properties in soil. Some studies about seasonal changes in MBC and SOC have been shown in **Table 2**. SOC changes in an ecosystem usually occur gradually and take a long time. However, soil microorganisms are very sensitive to any changes due to seasonal inputs of plant residues, structure, and growth of roots, chemical component released by root exudates, or decomposition of organic material inputs. Because the soil microbial activity has a direct impact on the stability and productivity of the ecosystem, microbial biomass provides very accurate and fast information about the quality of soil [55]. Few data is describing the seasonal variation of C and microbial carbon in the soil. If seasonal variation influences soil OC, environmental parameters that play an active role in this event should be determined, and their interaction with each other should be demonstrated in the same experimental unit over time.

Soil organic matter is considered to be composed of a large pool very slowly changing and protected [103, 104]. Also, it is believed that soil C and microbial activity is responsive and sensitive to any changes in terrestrial ecosystems. The amount of soil OC and MBC largely depends on the quality and quantity of litter input and microbial activity rate that could be affected by soil moisture, temperature, porosity, presence, and amount of nutrients. Climatic factors especially temperature and moisture are the most significant environmental factors affecting soil microbial biomass population and activity. Seasonal changes in soil temperature and humidity directly cause fluctuations of soil microbial biomass population and activity rates [43–45, 84–88]. In different types of microbial populations have the highest or lowest limits in which growth and activity decline [105]. Allen et al. [106] recommended that the determining effects of seasonal changes in the microbial activity of studies of spatial variability rarely consider sampling at the same time in a year. Seasonal effects in soil OC reveal numerous studies measuring basal respiration and microbial indexes, but total OC analysis is insufficient. Bolat et al. [76] found that seasonal fluctuations showed significant effects on microbial indexes such as MBC, MBN, and MBP in the forest floor and soil because of seasonal fluctuations that alter the climate and biogeochemical process of the soil. In the

		Organic carbon %				Cmic µg C g^{-1}				Ntop %			
	Seasons	Aut.	Win.	Spr.	Sum.	Aut.	Win.	Spr.	Sum.	Aut.	Win.	Spr.	Sum.
Studies	Tree species												
Barbhuiya et al. [88]	*Dipterocarpus macrocarpus, Shorea assamica, M. ferrea, T. nudiflora, Castanopsis indica and Vatica lanceaefolia*	1.33	1.65	1.51	—	1135	800	600	—	0.77	0.63	0.8	—
Devi and Yadava [80]	*Quercus serrata and Schima wallichii*	—	—	2.75–4.4		—	465.14	1182.6	738.32	—	—	0.39–0.54	
	Q.serrata and Lithocarpus dealbatus			2.6–4.34			382.58	740.73	392.92	—	—	0.33–0.50	
Muscolo and Sidari [116]	*Pinus laricio*	—	—	—	—	93	63	179	269	—	—	—	—
Bolat [45]	*Abies nordmanniana subsp. Bornmülleriana Mattf.*	6.08	5.35	6.06	5.21	1345	1016	714	845	0.36	0.32	0.34	0.32
	Fagus orientalis L.	3.75	3.75	3.26	4.15	650	567	517	629	0.23	0.24	0.2	0.26
	Mixed abies-fagus forest	3.33	3.33	3.01	2.28	844	476	505	757	0.22	0.19	0.17	0.16
Bolat et al. [76]	*Black locust*			0.64	0.72			311.97	483.34	0.17	0.21		
Siles et al. [117]	*Q. pubescens, Q. robur, F. sylvatica, Pinus sylvestris, Picea abies, Larix decidua, Fraxinus ornus, Ostrya carpinifolia*	29.25	—	18.19	—	—	—	—	—	1.06	—	0.78	—
Bargalia et al. [118]	*Oak forest*	2.99				554.3	540.7		545.7	0.21			
	Pine forest	1.96				467.3	446		451.3	0.09			
	Mixed oak-pine forest	5.3				728	710		716	0.32			
Babur [47]	*Cedrus libani*	4.93	4.39	4.78	4.48	807	401	635	486	0.405	0.303	0.393	0.361
	Fagus orientalis	5.36	5.2	4.62	5.58	691.8	547	539.99	658.08	0.34	0.223	0.315	0.353
	Black pine	4.56	4.62	4.33	4.45	659	252	309	590.2	0.27	0.179	0.239	0.23

Table 2.
Some studies about seasonal changes in MBC and SOC, TN.

same study, it was stated that microbial biomass reached the highest populations in the summer season.

In some of the studies mentioned below, the changes in soil organic carbon have been observed at different times of the year. Boerner et al. [107] studied on three mixed oak forest ecosystems in Ohio and found statistical differences in a variety of season and plant species. In another study in the Canadian prairie, four different samples were taken in spring, summer, autumn, and winter season [108]. In a study in Michigan, significant differences were found in the sampling in April and June which were 23% in a wheat field and 18% under poplar trees [109]. These studies indicate that seasonal changes are an important factor, but other factors may also be similarly involved, such as soil sampling technique and design and changes in soil water and temperature.

Seasonal changes in environmental conditions such as humidity and temperature facilitate the microbial biomass cycle, and therefore microbial biomass plays a crucial role in regulating nutrient uptake. Microbial biomass is considered dead if the soil substrate dries in summer or freezes in winter. Increases in microbial activity and population due to wetting and dissolution phenomena are attributed to the increase in available nutrients from dead microorganisms. Changes in soil temperature and humidity affect the C mineralization rate, the species structure of the microbial community, and the availability of nutrients from the soil solution [110, 111, 124, 125]. Carbon and microbial biomass carbon contents of soils formed under pure forest stands were investigated in research conducted in karstic areas of the Eastern Mediterranean region [47]. As a result of these investigations, it was stated that there was an increase in microbial biomass during the seasons where the soil temperature and humidity were optimum and that the seasons and plant species significantly affected the organic carbon and microbial biomass carbon contents of the soils (**Figure 6**) [47]. However, in another study conducted in the tropical Amazon rainforest, microbial biomass C indicates no significant seasonal changes [112]. Many researchers state that seasonal changes in microbial biomass are related to the water content and temperature conditions of the substrate [113–115]. In Spruce (*Picea rubens* Sarg.) forest, in a study carried out after heavy rains that occurred when the soil temperature reached +5° C, microbial biomass C was found to have a negative relationship with soil temperature, whereas microbial C, N, and P showed a positive relationship with soil moisture [116]. In another study, it was stated that the seasonal changes in microbial biomass were not only related to climatic conditions. Seasonal changes in microbial biomass may also be related to

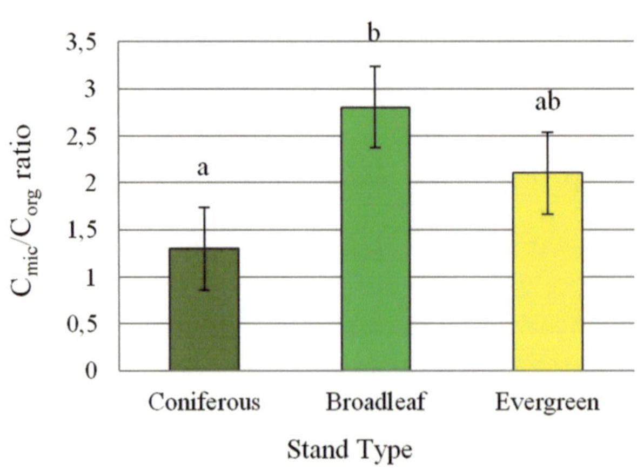

Figure 6.
The C_{mic}/C_{org} ratio determined in different stand types (changed from Bauhaus and Khanna, 1999).

changes in the amount of C that can be obtained from the amount of fine root, root secretions, and dead cover [111]. In various studies, it is emphasized that it is difficult to generalize the effect of tree species on microbial parameters.

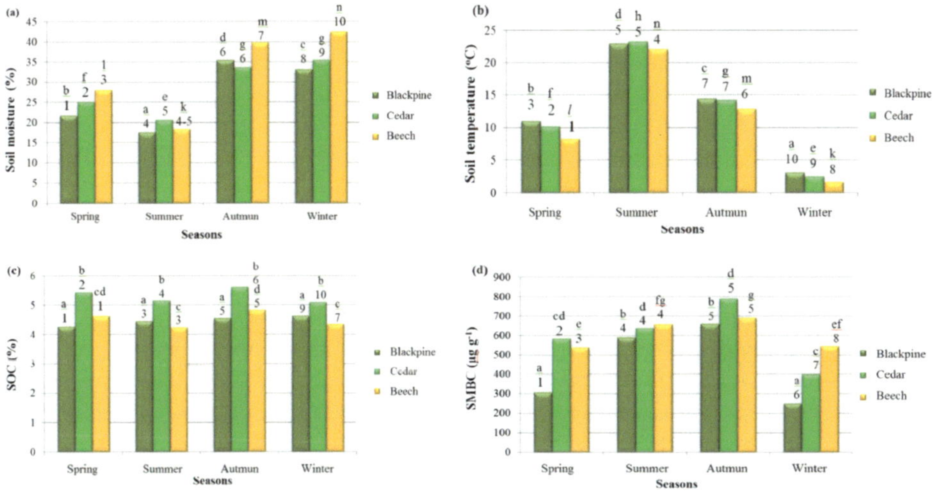

Figure 7.
(a) Moisture (%), (b) temperature (°C), (c) SOC and (d) SMBC mean values at soil samples. According to seasons n = 90 and tree species n = 120 total soil samples were analyzed. Different letters between seasons; the different numbers indicate differences between the tree species at the significance level of P < 0.05.

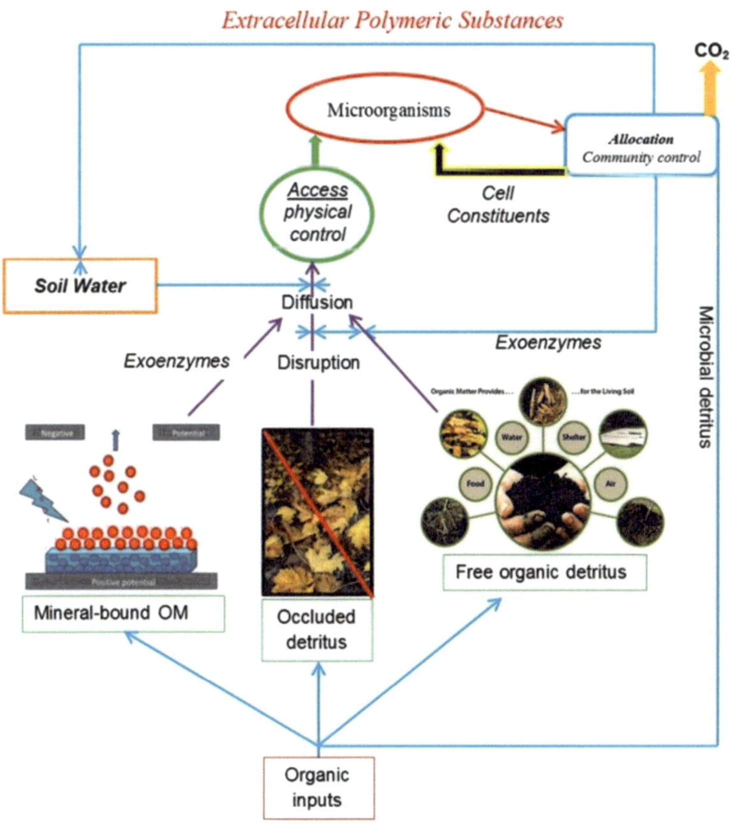

Figure 8.
Microbial C cycling the relative roles of physical access to soil C pools and of microbial allocation patterns in regulating overall soil C dynamics.

It is stated that C_{mic}/C_{org} percentage in leaf litter is higher in broadleaf forests (2.58%) than coniferous forests (1.27%), whereas it is stated that this value does not have a significant difference in evergreen forests (2.06%) (**Figure** 7). As a result of this study, it can be said that the litter quality of broadleaf species is better than the coniferous species or that the site factors of the broadleaf species are more suitable than the coniferous species for the microbial activity [111]. Similarly, Scheu and Parkinson [117] found that the amount of C_{mic} in the litter layer and the C_{mic}/C_{org} percentage were higher in the poplar stand than in the pine stands. The effective role of microorganisms in soil dynamics and the C cycle is shown in **Figure 8**.

Although soil microorganisms are a small part of soil organic material, it is an important factor that significantly and positively affects carbon storage in soil [36]. In addition to altering the physiology of microbial communities, changes in the availability of resources may indirectly affect microbial processes. The differences in substrates differ in the diversity of soil microorganism's community. These can lead to the supply of C, and nutrients from substrates are required for the productivity and biomass growth of forest ecosystems [110, 119–125], and also changes in sources have been shown to cause differences in microbial community composition [118, 126]. Changes in the composition of the microbial communities can significantly affect microbial processes, as certain enzymes are produced by specific groups of microorganisms [119, 120].

6. Conclusion

Consequently, any changes in quantity and quality of C and N in the soil directly influence on soil's biological characteristics. Furthermore, some various characteristics of soil such as temperature, moisture content, pH, silt, and clay content influence soil microbial activities [45–47]. Microbial microorganisms are very important in controlling nutrient dynamics and availability of soil ecosystem; on an annual basis, most of the nutrients for plants are maintained through mineralization of soil organic maters [105, 115]. Therefore, it is essential to investigate the seasonal changes of microbial activities and microbial biomass and the effects of seasonal changes (mostly temperature and water content) on them, to better understand the nutrient dynamics in tree species. The amounts of microbial population and activity significantly changed with the seasons and followed a sequence order (summer > autumn > spring > winter). In other words, microbial indexes such as MBC, MBN, and basal respiration rate in summer and autumn seasons are found to be higher than in spring and winter seasons.

This study illustrates that soil microbial community structure would vary with seasonal changes and tree species affect soil microbial community composition by changing the soil physicochemical properties.

Author details

Emre Babur* and Turgay Dindaroglu
Department of Forest Engineering, Kahramanmaraş Sütçü İmam University, Kahramanmaraş, Turkey

*Address all correspondence to: emrebabur@ksu.edu.tr

References

[1] Stockmann U, Adams MA, Crawford JW, Field DJ, et al. The knowns, known unknowns and unknowns of sequestration of soil organic carbon. Agriculture, Ecosystems and Environment. 2013;**164**:80-99

[2] FAO and ITPS. Status of the World's Soil Resources, Rome: s.n.; 2015

[3] Lal R, Follett RF. Soil Carbon Sequestration and the Greenhouse Effect. 2nd ed. Madison, Wisconsin, USA: Soil Science Society of America, Inc.; 2009

[4] Zeebe RE, Ridgwell A, Zachos JC. Anthropogenic carbon release rate unprecedented during the past 66 million years. Nature Geoscience. 2016; **9**:325-329

[5] Fahey TJ, Yavitt JB, Sherman RE, Maerz JC, Groffman PM, Fısk MC, et al. Earthworm effects on the incorporation of litter C and N into soil organic matter in a sugar maple forest. Ecological Applications. 2013;**23**(5):1185-1201

[6] Flato G, Marotzke J, Abiodun B, Braconnot P, Chou SC, Collins W, et al. Evaluation of climate models. In: Stocker TF, Qin D, Plattner G-K, Tignor M, Allen SK, Boschung J, et al., editors. Climate Change 2013: The Physical Science Basis. Contribution of Working Group I to the Fifth Assessment Report of the Intergovernmental Panel on Climate Change. Cambridge: Cambridge University Press; 2013

[7] Jaffe LS. Sources, characteristics, and fate of atmospheric carbon monoxide. Annals of the New York Academy of Sciences. 1970;**174**:76-88

[8] Lützow MV, Kögel-Knabner I, Ekschmitt K, Matzner E, Guggenberger G, Marschner B, et al. Stabilization of organic matter in temperate soils: Mechanisms and their relevance under different soil conditions —A review. European Journal of Soil Science. 2006;**57**:426-445

[9] Aertsen W, Kint V, Von Wilpert K, Zirlewagen D, Muys B, Van Orshoven J. Comparison of location-based, attribute-based and hybrid regionalization techniques for mapping forest site productivity. International Journal of Forestry Research. 2012; **85**(4):539-550

[10] NASA. 2009. https://www.nasa.gov/topics/earth/features/temp-analysis-2009.html [Accessed: 10 September 2019]

[11] Xu C, Guo L, Dou F, Ping C-L. Potential DOC production from sizefractionated Arctic tundra soils. Cold Regions Science and Technology. 2009;**55**:141-150

[12] Djukic I, Zehetner F, Tatzber M, Gerzabek MH. Soil organic-matter stocks and characteristics along an alpine elevation gradient. Journal of Plant Nutrition and Soil Science. 2010; **173**:30-38

[13] Franzluebbers AJ, Hons FM, Zuberer DA. Soil organic carbon, microbial biomass, and mineralizable carbon and nitrogen in sorghum. Soil Science Society of America Journal. 1995;**59**:460-466

[14] Bezdicek DF, Papendick RI, Lal R. Introduction: Importance of soil quality to health and sustainable land management. In: Doran JW, Jones AJ, editors. Methods of Assessing Soil Quality. Madison: SSSA Spec. Publ. 49; 1996. pp. 1-18

[15] Gulde S, Chung H, Amelung W, Chang C, Six J. Soil carbon saturation controls labile and stable carbon pool

dynamics. Soil Science Society of America Journal. 2008;**72**:605

[16] Russell MB, Fraver S, Aakala T, Gove JH, Woodall CW, D'Amato AW, et al. Quantifying carbon stores and decomposition in dead wood: A review. Forest Ecology and Management. 2015; **350**:107-128

[17] Kara Ö, Babur E, Altun L, Seyis M. Effects of afforestation on microbial biomass C and respiration in eroded soils of Turkey. Journal of Sustainable Forestry. 2016;**35**(1):385-396

[18] Magnússon RI, Tietema A, Cornelissen JHC, Hefting MM, Kalbitz K. Tamm review: Sequestration of carbon from coarse woody debris in forest soils. Forest Ecology and Management. 2016;**377**:1-15

[19] Hassink J. The capacity of soils to preserve organic C and N by their association with clay and silt particles. Plant and Soil. 2016;**191**:77-87

[20] Babur E. Effects of parent material on soil microbial biomass carbon and basal respiration within young afforested areas. Scaninavian Journal of Forest Research. 2019;**43**(2):94-101

[21] Batjes NH. Harmonized soil property values for broad-scale modelling (WISE30sec) with estimates of global soil carbon stocks. Geoderma. 2016;**269**:61-68

[22] Jobbágy EG, Jackson RB. The vertical distribution of soil organic carbon and its relation to climate and vegetation. Ecological Applications. 2000;**10**:423-436

[23] Churchman GJ. Game changer in soil science: Functional role of clay minerals in soil. Journal of Plant Nutrition and Soil Science. 2018;**181**: 99-103

[24] Gabarron-Galeote MA, Trigalet S, van Wesemael B. Effect of land abandonment on soil organic carbon fractions along a Mediterranean precipitation gradient. Geoderma. 2015;**249–250**:69-78

[25] Schimel JP, Schaffer SM. Microbial control over carbon cycling in soil. Frontiers in Microbiology. 2012;**348**(3): 1-11

[26] Trumbore SE, Czimczik CI. An uncertain future for soil carbon. Science. 2008;**321**(5895):1455-1456

[27] Gärdenäs AI, Ågren GI, Bird JA, et al. Knowledge gaps in soil carbon and nitrogen interactions – From molecular to global scale. Soil Biology and Biochemistry. 2011;**43**(4):702-717

[28] Link 1. http://www.ridgedaleperma culture.com/blog/we-like-well-engineered-stuff2 Soil sample under microscope mauby.com [Accessed: 28 September 2019]

[29] Lal R. Why carbon sequestration in agricultural soils. In: Kimble JM, Lal R, Follett RF, editors. Agricultural Practices and Policies for Carbon Sequestration in Soil. Boca Raton: Lewis Publishers; 2002. pp. 21-30

[30] Jandl R, Lindner M, Vesterdal L, Bauwens B, Baritz R, Hagedorn F, et al. How strongly can forest management influence soil carbon sequestration? Geoderma. 2007;**137**:253-268

[31] Blanco JA, Lo YH, Welham C, Larson B. Productivity of forest ecosystems. In: Innes J, Tikina A, editors. Sustainable Forest Management: From Principles to Practice. London: Earthscan; 2017

[32] Seely B, Welham C, Blanco JA. Towards the application of soil organic matter as an indicator of ecosystem productivity: Deriving thresholds, developing monitoring systems, and evaluating practices. Ecological Indicators. 2010;**10**:999-1008

[33] Doran JW, Parkin TB. Defining and assessing soil quality. In: Doran JW, Coleman DC, Bezdick DF, Stewart BA, editors. Defining Soil Quality for a Sustainable Environment. Vol. 35. Madison, WI, USA: Soil Science Society of America Inc.; 1994. pp. 3-21

[34] Morris DM, Kimmins JP, Duckert DR. The use of soil organic matter as a criterion of the relative sustainability of forest management alternatives: A modelling approach using FORECAST. Forest Ecology and Management. 1997;**94**:61-78

[35] Prescott CE, Maynard DG, Laiho R. Humus in northern forests: Friend or foe? Forest Ecology and Management. 2000;**133**:23-36

[36] Jenkinson DS, Ladd JN. Microbial biomass in soil measurement and turnover. In: Paul EA, Ladd JN, editors. Soil Biochemistry. Vol. 5. New York: Marcel Dekker Inc; 1981. pp. 415-471

[37] Henrot J, Robertson GP. Vegetation removal in two soils of the humid tropics: Effect on microbial biomass. Soil Biology and Biochemistry. 1994;**26**(1): 111-116

[38] Mahía J, Pérez-Ventura L, Cabaneiro A, Díaz-Raviña M. Soil microbial biomass under pine forests in the North-Western Spain: Influence of stand age, site index and parent material. Forest Systems. 2006;**15**(2): 152-159

[39] Kara Ö, Bolat İ. Soil microbial biomass C and N changes in relation to forest conversion in the northwestern Turkey. Land Degradation and Development. 2008a;**19**(4):421-428

[40] Alvarez E, Torrado VM, Fernandez Marcos ML, Diaz-Ravia M. Microbial biomass and activity in a forest soil under different tree species. Electronic Journal of Environmental, Agricultural and Food Chemistry. 2009; **8**(9):878-887

[41] Tolunay D. Carbon concentrations of tree components, forest floor and understorey in young Pinus sylvestris stands in North-Western Turkey. Scandinavian Journal of Forest Research. 2009;**24**(5):394-402

[42] Çömez A. Determination of Carbon Sequestration in Scots Pine (Pinus sylvestris L.) Stands on Sündiken Mountain-Eskişehir. Eskişehir (in Turkish): Research Institute for Forest Soil and Ecology Press; 2012

[43] Vinisa S, Claudia H, Jorge DE. Soil C and N dynamics in primary and secondary seasonally dry tropical forests in Mexico. Applied Soil Ecology. 2005; **29**:282-289

[44] Patel K, Nirmal Kumar JIN, Kumar R, Kumar BR. Seasonal and temporal variation in soil microbial biomass C, N and P in different types land uses of dry deciduous forest ecosystem of Udaipur, Rajasthan, Western India. Applied Ecology and Environmental Research. 2010;**8**(4): 377-390

[45] Bolat I. Seasonal changes in microbial biomass carbon (cmic), nitrogen (nmic), phosphorus (pmic), and microbial respiration of forest floor and top soil under beech, fir and mixed fir-beech forest stands [thesis]. Graduate School of Natural and Applied Sciences, Department of Forestry Engineering. Turkey: Bartın University (in Turkish); 2011

[46] Kara Ö, Bolat İ, Çakıroğlu K, Şentürk M. Litter decomposition and microbial biomass in temperate forests in northwestern Turkey. Journal of Soil Science and Plant Nutrition. 2014;**14**(1): 31-41

[47] Babur E. Determination of carbon-nitrogen stock in forest floor and soil of even-aged black pine, lebanon cedar and oriental beech forest in karstic ecosystems; monitoring of seasonal

changes in some microbial properties [PhD. thesis]. Graduate School of Natural and Applied Sciences, Department of Forestry Engineering. Turkey: Kahramanmaraş Sütçü İmam University (in Turkish); 2018

[48] Brookes P. The soil microbial biomass: Concept, measurement and applications in soil ecosystem research. Microbes and Environments. 2001; **16**(3):131-140

[49] Anderson TH, Domsch KH. Application of eco-physiological quotients (qCO2, and qD) on microbial biomasses from soils of different cropping histories. Soil Biology and Biochemistry. 1990;**22**:251-255

[50] Sparling GP. Soil microbial biomass, activity and nutrient cycling as indicators of soil health. In: Pankhurst C, Doube BM, Gupta VVSR, editors. Biological Indicators of Soil Health. Wallingford: CAB International; 1997. pp. 97-119

[51] Schoenholtz SH, Van Miegroet H, Burger JA. A review of chemical and physical properties as indicators of forest soil quality: Challenges and opportunities. Forest Ecology and Management. 2000;**138**:335-356

[52] Gregorich EG, Liang BC, Drury CF, Mackenzie AF, McGill WB. Elucidation of the source and turnover of water soluble and microbial biomass carbon in agricultural soils. Soil Biology and Biochemistry. 2000;**32**:581-587

[53] Haney RL, Franzluebbers AJ, Hons FM, Hossner LR, Zuberer DA. Molar concentration of K2SO4 and soil pH effect estimation of extractable C with chloroform fumigation extraction. Soil Biology and Biochemistry. 2001;**33**: 1501-1507

[54] Rice CW, Smith MS, Blevins RL. Soil nitrogen availability after long-term continuous no-tillage and conventional tillage corn production. Soil Science Society of America Journal. 1986;**50**: 1206-1210

[55] Smith LJ. Papen-dick. Soil organic matter dynamics and crop residue management. In: Metting B, editor. Soil Microbial Ecology. New York: Marcel Dekker; 1993

[56] Powlson DS, Jenkinson DS. A comparison of the organic-matter, biomass, adenosine-triphosphate and mineralizable nitrogen contents of ploughed and direct-drilled soils. Journal of Agricultural Science. 1981;**97**: 713-721

[57] Powlson DS, Brookes PC, Jenkinson DS. Measurement of soil microbial biomass provides an early indication of changes in total soil organic matter due to straw incorporation. Soil Biology and Biochemistry. 1987;**19**:159-164

[58] Pankhurst CE, Doube BM, Gupta VVSR. Biological indicators of soil health: Synthesis. In: Pankhurst CE, Doube BM, Gupta VVSR, editors. Biological Indicators of Soil Health. Wallingford, UK: CAB International; 1997. pp. 419-435

[59] Nielsen MN, Winding A. Microorganisms as Indicators of Soil Health. National Environmental Research Institute, Technical Report No. 388, Denmark 1–84; 2002

[60] Insam H, Parkinson D, Domsch KH. Influence of macroclimate on soil microbial biomass. Soil Biology and Biochemistry. 1989;**21**(19890):211-221

[61] Arunachalam A. Role of microbial biomass in soil nutrient dynamics along a jhum cycle gradient. Journal of Tropical Forest Science. 2003;**15**(2): 279-288

[62] Liebig MA, Tanaka DL, Wienhold BJ. Tillage and cropping

effects on soil quality indicators in the northern Great Plains. Soil & Tillage Research. 2004;**78**:131-141

[63] Azam F, Farooq S, Lodhi A. Microbial biomass in agricultural soils-determination, synthesis, dynamics and role in plant nutrition. Pakistan Journal of Biological Sciences. 2003;**6**: 629-639

[64] Wardle DA. A comparative assessment of factors which influence microbial biomass carbon and nitrogen levels in soil. Biological Reviews. 1992; **67**:321-358

[65] Canarini A, Kaiser C, Merchant A, Richter A, Wanek W. Root exudation of primary metabolites: Mechanisms and their roles in plant responses to environmental stimuli. Frontiers in Plant Science. 2019;**10**:157

[66] Dinesh R, Srinivasan V, Hamza S, Parthasarathy VA, Aipe KC. Physico-chemical, biochemical and microbial properties of the rhizospheric soils of tree species used as supports for black pepper cultivation in the humid tropics. Geoderma. 2010;**158**:252-258

[67] Cao D, Shi F, Koike T, Lu Z, Sun Z. Halophyte plant communities affecting enzyme activity and microbes in saline soils of the Yellow River Delta in China. CLEAN – Soil, Air, Water. 2014;**42**: 1433-1440

[68] Chaudhary DR, Gautam RK, Yousuf B, Mishra A, Jha B. Nutrients, microbial community structure and functional gene abundance of rhizosphere and bulk soils of halophytes. Applied Soil Ecology. 2015; **91**:16-26

[69] Brimecombe MJ, De Leij FA, Lynch JA. The effect of root exudates on rhizosphere microbial populations. In: Pinton R, Varanini Z, Nannipieri P, editors. The Rhizosphere: Biochemistry and Organic Substances at the Soil–Plant Interface. New York: Marcel Dekker Inc.; 2001. pp. 95-104

[70] Barness G, Zaragoza SR, Shmueli I, Steinberger Y. Vertical distribution of a soil microbial community as affected by plant ecophysiological adaptation in a desert system. Microbial Ecology. 2009; **57**:36-49

[71] Mishra RR, Swain MR, Dangar TK, Thatoi H. Diversity and seasonal fluctuation of predominant microbial communities in Bhitarkanika, a tropical mangrove ecosystem in India. Revista de Biología Tropical. 2012;**60**: 909-924

[72] Richards AE, Forrester DI, Bauhus J, Scherer-Lorenzen M. The influence of mixed tree plantations on the nutrition of individual species: A review. Tree Physiology. 2010;**30**:1192-1208

[73] Malchair S, Carnol M. Microbial biomass and C and N transformation in forest floors under European beech, sessile oak, Norway spruce and Douglas-fir at four temperate forest sites. Soil Biology and Biochemistry. 2009;**41**: 831-839

[74] Morrissey EM, Gillespie JL, Morina JC, Franklin RB. Salinity affects microbial activity and soil organic matter content in tidal wetlands. Global Change Biology. 2014;**20**:1351-1362

[75] Singh K. Microbial and enzyme activities of saline and sodic soils. Land Degradation and Development. 2015;**27**: 706-718

[76] Bolat İ, Şensoy H, Özer D. Short-term changes in microbial biomass and activity in soils under black locust trees (Robinia pseudoacacia L.) in the northwest of Turkey. Journal of Soils and Sediments. 2015;**15**:2189-2198

[77] Khan B, Ablimit A, Mahmood R, Qasim M. Robinia pseudoacacia leaves improve soil physical and chemical

properties. Journal of Arid Land. 2010; **2**(4):266-271

[78] Wang B, Liu G, Xue S. Effect of black locust (Robinia pseudoacacia) on soil chemical and microbiological properties in the eroded hilly area of China's loess plateau. Environment and Earth Science. 2012;**65**(3):597-607

[79] Vlachodimos K, Papatheodorou EM, Diamantopoulos J, Monokrousos N. Assessment of Robinia pseudoacacia cultivations as a restoration strategy for reclaimed mine spoil heaps. Environmental Monitoring and Assessment. 2013;**185**(8):6921-6932

[80] Devi NB, Yadava PS. Seasonal dynamics in soil microbial biomass C, N and P in a mixed-oak forest ecosystem of Manipur, north-East India. Applied Soil Ecology. 2006;**31**:220-227

[81] Edwards KA, Meculloch JF, Kershaw GP, Jefferies RL. Soil microbial and nutrient dynamics in a wet arctic sedge meadow in late winter and early spring. Soil Biology and Biochemistry. 2006;**38**(9):2843-2851

[82] Joergensen RG, Anderson TH, Wolters V. Carbon and nitrogen relationships in the microbial biomass of soils in beech (Fagus sylvatica L.) forests. Biology and Fertility of Soils. 1995;**19**:141-147

[83] Kara Ö, Bolat İ, Çakıroğlu K, Öztürk M. Plant canopy effects on litter accumulation and soil microbial biomass in two temperate forests. Biology and Fertility of Soils. 2008;**45**(2):193-198

[84] Yang JC, Insam H. Microbial biomass and relative contributions of bacteria and fungi in beneath tropical rain forest, Hainan Island. Chinese Journal of Tropical Ecology. 1991;**7**: 385-395

[85] Maithani K, Tripathi RS, Arunachalam A, Pandey HN. Seasonal dynamics of microbial biomass C, N and P during regrowth of a disturbed subtropical humid forest in Northeast India. Applied Soil Ecology. 1996;**4**: 31-37

[86] Lipson DA, Schmidt SK, Monson RK. Links between microbial population dynamics and plant nitrogen availability in an alpine ecosystem. Ecology. 1999;**80**(5):1623-1631

[87] Chen CR, Condron LM, Davis MR, Sherlock RR. Seasonal changes in soil phosphorus and associated microbial properties under adjacent grassland and forest in New Zealand. Forest Ecology and Management. 2003;**177**:539-557

[88] Barbhuiya AR, Arunachalam A, Pandeyb HN, Arunachalam K, Khan ML. Dynamics of soil microbial biomass C, N and P in disturbed and undisturbed stands of a tropical wet-evergreen forest. European Journal of Soil Biology. 2004;**40**:113-121

[89] Zhou GM, Xu JM, Jiang PK. Effect of management practices on seasonal dynamics of organic carbon in soils under bamboo plantations. Pedosphere. 2006;**16**(4):525-531

[90] Kramer S, Green DM. Acid and alkaline phosphatase dynamics and their relationship to soil microclimate in a semiarid woodland. Soil Biology and Biochemistry. 2000;**32**:179-188

[91] Dick RP. Enzyme activities as integrative indicators of soil health. In: Pankhurst C, Doube BM, Gupta VVSR, editors. Biological Indicators of Soil Health. Wallingford: CAB International; 1997. pp. 121-156

[92] Doran JW, Safley M. Defining and assessing soil health and sustainable productivity. In: Pankhurst C, Doube BM, Gupta VVSR, editors. Biological Indicators of Soil Health. Wallingford: CAB International; 1997. pp. 1-28

[93] Marinari S, Mancinelli R, Campiglia E, Grego S. Chemical and biological indicators of soil quality in organic and conventional farming systems in Central Italy. Ecological Indicators. 2006;**6**(4):701-711

[94] Zhu B, Li Z, Li P, Liu G, Xue S. Soil erodibility, microbial biomass, and physical–chemical property changes during long-term natural vegetation restoration: A case study in the loess plateau. Chinese Journal of Ecology. 2010;**25**(3):531-541

[95] Davidson EA, Janssens IA. Temperature sensitivity of soil carbon decomposition and feedbacks to climate change. Nature. 2006;**440**:165-173

[96] Chapin FS, Mooney HA, Matson PA. Principles of Terrestrial Ecosystem Ecology. New York: Springer-Verlag; 2002

[97] Schmidt MWI, Torn MS, Abiven S, Dittmar T, Guggenberger G, Janssens IA, et al. Persistence of soil organic matter as an ecosystem property. Nature. 2011;**478**:49-56

[98] Olander LP, Vitousek PM. Regulation of soil phosphatase and chitinase activity by N and P availability. Biogeochemistry. 2000;**49**: 175-190

[99] Allison SD, Vitousek PM. Responses of extracellular enzymes to simple and complex nutrient inputs. Soil Biology & Biochemistry. 2005;**37**:937-944

[100] Hernandez DL, Hobbie SE. The effects of substrate composition, quantity and diversity on microbial activity. Plant and Soil. 2010;**335**: 397-411

[101] Winding A, Hund-Rinke K, Rutgers M. The use of microorganisms in ecological soil classification and assessment concepts. Ecotoxicology and Environmental Safety. 2005;**62**:230-248

[102] Insam H, Mitchell CC, Dormaar JF. Relationship of soil microbial biomass and activity with fertilization practice and crop yield of three ultisols. Soil Biology and Biochemistry. 1991;**23**(5): 459-464

[103] Fierer N, Grandy AS, Six J, Paul EA. Searching for unifying principles in soil ecology. Soil Biology and Biochemistry. 2009;**41**:2249-2256

[104] Kiem R, Kögel-Knabner I. Contribution of lignin and polysaccharides to the refractory carbon pool in C-depleted arable soils. Soil Biology and Biochemistry. 2003;**35**: 101-118

[105] Paul EA, Clark FE. Soil Microbiology and Biochemistry. San Diego, Californina, USA: Academic Press; 1996. p. 340

[106] Allen DE, Pringle MJ, Page KL, Dalal RC. A review of sampling designs for the measurement of soil organic carbon in Australian grazing lands. Rangeland Journal. 2010;**32**:227-246

[107] Boerner REJ, Brinkman JA, Smith A. Seasonal variations in enzyme activity and organic carbon in soil of a burned and unburned hardwood forest. Soil Biology and Biochemistry. 2005;**37**: 1419-1426

[108] Dormaar JF, Johnston A, Smoliak S. Seasonal variation in chemical characteristics of soil organic matter of grazed and ungrazed mixed prairie and fescue grassland. Journal of Range Management. 1977;**30**:195-198

[109] Stoyan H, De-Polli H, Bohm S, Robertson GP, Paul EA. Spatial heterogeneity of soil respiration and related properties at the plant scale. Plant and Soil. 2000;**222**:203-214

[110] Zogg GP, Zak DR, Ringelberg DB, MacDonald NW, Pregitzer KS, White DC. Compositional and functional shifts in microbial

communities related to soil warming. Soil Science Society of America Journal. 1997;**61**:475-481

[111] Bauhus J, Khanna PK. The significance of microbial biomass in forest soils. In: Rastin N, Bauhus J, editors. Going Underground - Ecological Studies in Forest Soils. Trivandrum, India: Research Signpost; 1999. pp. 77-110

[112] Luizao RCC, Bonde RA, Rosswall T. Seasonal variation of soil microbial biomass: The effect of clear felling in a tropical rain forest and establishment of pasture in the Central Amazon. Soil Biology and Biochemistry. 1992;**24**: 805-813

[113] Entry JA, Stark NM, Loewenstein H. Effect of timber harvesting on microbial biomass fluxes in a northern Rocky Mountain forest soil. Canadian Journal of Forest Research. 1986;**16**:1076-1081

[114] Santruckova H. Microbial biomass, activity and soil respiration in relation to secondary succession. Pedobiologia. 1992;**36**:341-350

[115] Diaz-Ravina M, Acea MJ, Carballas T. Seasonal changes in microbial biomass and nutrient flush in forest soils. Biology and Fertility of Soils. 1995;**19**:220-226

[116] Christ MJ, David MB, McHale PJ, McLaughlin JW, Mitchell MJ, Rustad LE, et al. Microclimatic control of microbial C, N, and P pools in Spodosol Oa-horizons. Canadian Journal of Forest Research. 1997;**27**:1914-1921

[117] Scheu S, Parkinson D. Successional changes in microbial biomass, respiration and nutrient status during litter decompo-sition in an aspen and pine forest. Biology and Fertility of Soils. 1995;**19**:327-332

[118] Gusewell S, Gessner MO. N:P ratios influence litter decomposition and colonization by fungi and bacteria in microcosms. Functional Ecology. 2009; **23**:211-219

[119] Fierer N, Lauber CL, Ramirez KS, Zaneveld J, Bradford MA, Knight R. Comparative metagenomic, phylogenetic and physiological analyses of soil microbial communities across nitrogen gradients. ISME Journal. 2012; **6**:1007-1017

[120] Balser TC, Firestone MK. Linking microbial community composition and soil processes in a California annual grassland and mixed-conifer forest. Biogeochemistry. 2005;**73**:395-415

[121] Schimel JP, Schaffer SM. Microbial control over carbon cycling in soil. Frontiers in Microbiology. 2012;**3**(348): 348

[122] Arunachalam A, Arunachalam K. Influence of gap size and soil properties on microbial biomass in a subtropical humid forest of north-East India. Plant and Soil. 2000;**223**:185-193

[123] Muscolo A. Sidari. M. Seasonal fluctuations in soil phenolics of a coniferous forest: Effects on seed germination of different coniferous species. Plant and Soil. 2006;**284**:305-318

[124] Siles JA, Cajthaml T, Filipova A, Minerbi S, Margesin R. Altitudinal, seasonal and interannual shifts in microbial communities and chemical composition of soil organic matter in alpine forest soils. Soil Biology & Biochemistry. 2017;**112**:1-13

[125] Bargalia K, Manrala V, Padaliaa K, Bargalia SS, Upadhyayb VP. Effect of vegetation type and season on microbial biomass carbon in central Himalayan forest soils, India. Catena. 2018;**171**: 125-135

[126] Waldrop MP, Zak DR, Sinsabaugh RL. Microbial community response to nitrogen deposition in northern forest ecosystems. Soil Biology & Biochemistry. 2004;**36**:1443-1451

Chapter 8

Sugar Industry Wastes as Wealth of Organic Carbon for Soil

Anbalagan Krishnaveni, Sivakumar Chinnasamy, Jamuna Elumalai and Pandiyan Muthaiyan

Abstract

The organic carbon management in the soil and its relationship with soil physiochemical and biological characteristics to increase the crop productivity have been described based on the byproducts of sugarcane. In this chapter, the available information on the nutrient content especially the organic carbon of various by-products of sugarcane, paves the way for incorporation of waste materials and its compost for improving the soil fertility by soil scientists and agronomists, and further, the ecologists will realize the importance of sugarcane waste and its meritorious characteristics of toxic residue free soil and food products in addition to reducing the emission of greenhouse gases to the atmosphere, especially methane and nitrous oxides due to applied of synthetic fertilizer in the cultivating field. We have compiled the information on relationship between organic carbon and soil characteristic, factors responsible for depletion of soil organic carbon and its management. The composting process for sugarcane press mud, bagasse, and trash to produce nutrient-rich manure for soil fertility management and its value on saving the purchase of chemical fertilizer leads to easy adoption of organic farming. Overall, we emphasized the importance of waste products of sugarcane and it's nutritive value to increase the soil fertility, crop productivity, and farm income.

Keywords: nutrient composition, press mud, bagasse, molasses, microbial status, enzyme activity

1. Introduction

The organic carbon is essential to activate the physical, chemical, and biological components formation in the soil. The organic carbon is a perennial element because all macro- and micronutrients utilized by flora and fauna are decomposed and finally deposited as carbon-rich organic matter, humus, fossil fuel, etc., in the soil layers. But, the formation and deposition processes have become very low due to intensive cropping system, monocropping system without incorporation of leguminous crops as a sole crop or intercrop, lack of in situ crop residue recycling, poor application of organic manures, leaching of soil top fertile layer due to improper soil conservation measures, and excessive use of chemical fertilizers and other socio-economic factors. In this world, enormous quantity of organic by-products of animal and plant based are available to enrich or sustain the carbon level in the soil. There are many agro-based industries, especially the sugarcane-based sugar industry is widely located and generates different types of by-products like press mud, molasses, bagasse, etc., during the production of crystal sugar for commercial purpose. These by-products are not being utilized as organic manure to the soil due to lack of awareness of its nutrient's richness, particularly organic carbon and other nutrients. Instead, these by-products have been heaped or improperly disposed in and around the industrial factories resulting major health impacts to local residents and livestock are in addition to soil and air pollution. The sugarcane-based by-products contain lignocellulosic compounds that are the main source of carbon through microbial decomposition. In turn, the organic carbon is very essential for the microbial nitrogen mineralization and also crucial for the solubilization of fixed nutrients, particularly phosphorus and potassium in the clay particles of different soil types. Overall, the organic carbon is the heart of the soil for its nature to activate the action of biotic and abiotic components in the soil ecosystem. The knowledge on status, importance, and sources of organic carbon in the soil is very important to manage the continuously decreasing the organic carbon content, which ultimately affect the floral biodiversity of the soil.

1.1 Status of soil organic carbon in different types of soil

The status of organic carbon in the soil varies according to the soil organic matter content and its nature of origin, i.e., plants, animals, minerals, etc. The organic carbons will be estimated easily based on the soil organic matter status. In general, the organic carbon content of the soil is 1.72 times lesser than the soil organic matters. Overall, the higher end of soil organic carbon ranges between 0.1 and 10.0 per cent in various types of soil in the different region. its productivity is assessed based on physical, chemical, and biological traits in addition to floral and faunal diversity. The biodiversity of the soil is directly connected to the soil organic carbon or fertility status and also crop productivity. The soil nutrient status is very important for the growth and development of crop for different stages like seedling, vegetative, reproductive, and maturity to complete its life cycle and finally to attain its senescence. If the soil is having major and micronutrient deficiency means it will be shown on the plant as nutritional deficiency symptoms due to improper physiological activities and to some extent it will invite different pest and pathogens attack, which result to lowest yields when compared to its maximum yield potentiality. The organic carbon content in the different ecosystems like terrestrial, aquatic, grassland, forest, etc., contain different levels with maximum of 60 %. The organic carbon in the organic matter in the 1 m of Earth soil is 2200 Gt. Soil is a mother to flora, fauna, and human being through its sacrifices as habitat, food generator in the form of fruits, vegetables, grains, and medicines to cure different diseases in addition to maintaining the ecological and climate balance of the Earth.

1.2 Formula for estimating soil organic carbon

Soil organic carbon available in different pools is 15–225 t Carbon per ha in the 0–30 cm soil layer. The formation of soil organic carbon is due to mineralization of carbon and nutrients [1]. The total mass of organic matter, i.e., 58%, exists as carbon. To measure the total organic carbon (%), the conversion factor is 1.72 or 100/58; hence, organic matter (%) = total organic carbon (%) $\times$ 1.72. This conversion factor will differ from soil to soil. But, the value 1.72 gives reasonable value of soil organic matter.

1.3 Importance of organic carbon in the soil

The physicochemical and biological properties in the soil are either directly or indirectly depending on the soil organic carbon for its formation and reaction.

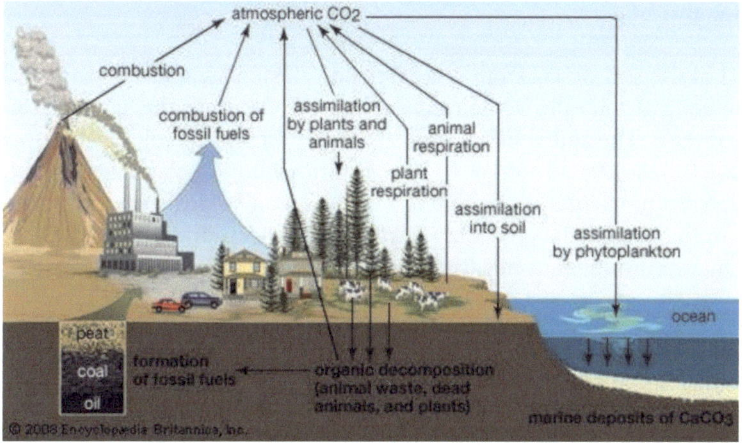

Figure 1.
Flow carbon in the soil ecosystem depending on many factors, for example changing climate, land use, soil layer in the critical zone (editors of Encyclopedia Britannica).

The soil organic carbon is calculated and expressed in the unit percentage (%). The minimum level of organic carbon in the soil plays a major role in the activation of soil chemical reactions and microbial growth and development. The major source of organic carbons is from organic matter of either plant or animal origin. Generally, the differences of soil organic matter, inorganic soil carbon, and organic carbon differ through its persistence in the soil. **Figure 1** indicates that the particulate organic carbons comes from fresh leaf residues and living organism with labile nature of 1–5 years. The humus organic carbon has 20–40 years of association with the soil organic matter of soil, whereas the resistant organic carbon from humus and charcoal has 500–1000 years of bond with the soil organic matter. Soil functions are the important function on Earth's land zone to support the living and nonliving things formation and disintegrate into different organic and inorganic compounds to supply energy and nutrient to the flora and fauna species. The carbon is the basic element for the entire living organism to build its body mass and further multiplication. The flow carbon in the soil ecosystem depends on many factors, for example, changing climate, land use, and soil layer in the critical zone (**Figure 1**).

2. Soil physical properties

The physical properties are mainly the structure and texture of soil. It mainly depends on size of soil particles bond with particulate organic carbon of clay particles of different types of involves in the structural stability of soil from silt to sand. The particle size of the soil varies from coarse sand (2.0–0.2 mm), fine sand (0.2–0.02 mm), silt (0.02–0.002 mm), and fine clay (<0.002). The particle density of the good soil are 2.65 mega grams per cubic meter.

2.1 Soil color

The physical property like color of the soil indicates the organic carbon content, for example, the soil color is black means it has more organic carbon, which absorbs maximum solar radiation and paves for long-time photosynthesis that results in more crop productivity. The red soil shows rich in iron compounds, whereas the light yellow color indicate the iron oxidized soil. The light blue color soil is water logged soils.

2.2 Soil pH and EC

The pH of the soil varies from scale 0 to 14. The acid soil indicates the pH from 0 to 6.5. The neutral soil falls in the range of 6.5–7.5, whereas the alkaline soils has the pH value of >7.5. The soil is EC of indicate soil indicator of soluble salts present in the soil, 0–1.0, 1.1–3.0, >3.1 ds m^{-1}. The montmorillonite clay has the highest ion change capacity particularly positive ion exchange. The positive and negative ions exchange in the outside layer of clay particles. The iron-and aluminum-rich soil show the maximum level of negative ion exchange.

2.3 Soil particles

The soil particles will be classified into microaggregates like 2–20 and 20–250 mm and macro aggregates >250. Microaggregates diameters (2–20 mm) were formed through flocculation of silt clay particles. The negatively charged clay particles are increased through addition of exchangeable calcium cation and also the available trivalent aluminum cation. The microaggregates (20–250 mm) were formed initially from the products available through decomposition of organic debris.

The soil macroaggregates (>250 mm) contains primary particles, whereas the microaggregates are associated with plant root mycorrhizae and particulate organic matter and its stability maintained by soil management. The water holding capacity, porosity, bulk density, and strength of the soil depend on the stability of the soil aggregate. The soil organic carbon of the soil is decreasing from 1.5 to 1.2%, which means that the stability of micro- and macro aggregates of soil is also decreasing simultaneously. About 2% level of soil organic carbon is required to stabilize the soil micro- and macro aggregates [2]. The maximum soil organic carbon for the soil aggregates stability is 3.2–4.0% [3]. The soil particles aggregates stability does not reach a limit; the process of stability will increase with increase in soil organic matter content of the soil due to microbial decomposition [4].

3. Chemical properties

The chemical properties of the soil will influence the certain functions of the floras. The organic carbon contributes to the chemical elements cation exchange capacity and also enhances buffer capacity in accordance to changing pH of the soil. Chemical functions of the organic carbon contribute to the chemical elements cation exchange capacity and also enhance buffer capacity in accordance to changing pH of the soil. The cations and anions' complexes reduce the availability of toxic cation like Al_3^+ in the soil solution. The cations and anions' complexes reduce the availability of toxic cation like Al_3^+ in the soil solution. To estimate the capacity of soil carbon, fractions to undertake some of the functions vary with different soil types. The main organic carbon sources in the soil are humic and fulvic acids, which are holding highest chemical activity, whereas the particulate organic carbon is mainly involving in soil aggregates stability and texture. In general, the standard amount of the soil carbon compounds are essential for the soil functions like water holding capacity and enzymatic microbial activity for the mineralization of nutritive elements. Krull et al. [5] reported that the importance of the different organic carbon fractions for its role in plant physiological functions varies with respect to different soil types. The soil organic matter paves the importance functions of provide cation exchange capacity in sandy type of soil. The most important function

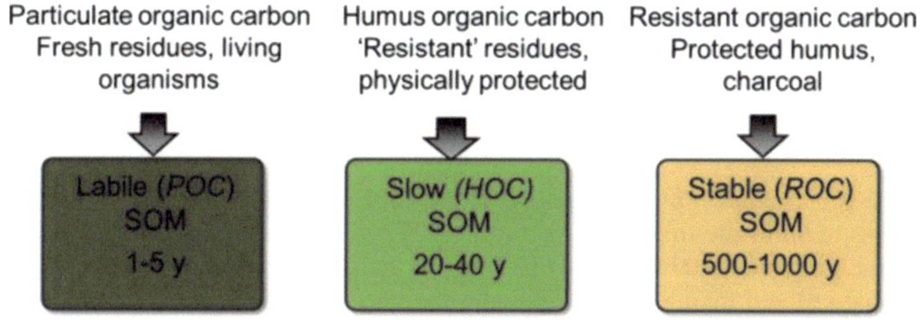

Figure 2.
Different types of carbon and its longevity with soil organic matter. (University of Minnesota Extension Publication WW-07402).

the need for soil organic matter to provide a food and energy source for the microbial populations is needed in all soils, regardless of clay content or texture

3.1 Soil organic matter

Soil organic matter in the soil comprises of all the organic materials available in soils through natural or external application. The natural sources include microbial organisms, flora and fauna, particulate organic matter, humus, charred organic materials, and charcoal. The definition of soil organic matter excludes larger than 2 mm size organic materials [6].

3.2 Soil organic carbon

Soil organic matter consists of carbon, hydrogen, oxygen, nitrogen, phosphorus, and sulfur. The soil organic matter has been actually determined analytically based on the level of soil organic carbon. The common conversion factor is 1.72. The content of soil organic matter will be calculated through the soil organic carbon multiplied with 1.72 [6]. The different types of carbon and its longevity with soil organic matters are shown in **Figure 2**.

3.3 Inorganic soil carbon

The inorganic carbon will originate in arid soils in combination with more mineral materials like basalts, limestone, and calcium, and is also formed from magnesium carbonate or dolomite. The inorganic carbon is not counted in the soil organic carbon level. The inorganic carbon will not contribute the soil organic matter [7].

4. Biological functions

The biological function of carbon-containing organic matters provides a major carbon, hydrogen, and nitrogen sources of energy to microorganisms for its metabolism. The microbial load and its activity are very essential for the biological processes like nutrient elements mineralization, decomposition of organic residues, and also solubilization of fixed nutrients in clay particles of the soil. The microbial action in the soil is highly dependent on the organic carbon through organic matter decomposition which further involves in the nutrient recycling in the crop land ecosystem (**Table 1**). The different microbial categories are involving in different function for the nutrients uptake by plants.

4.1 Factors influencing the organic carbon content in the soil

The organic carbon balance is very important for initiation of all the physical processes to build the soil structure and texture, which are essential for plant growth and further establishment. The organic carbon balance of the soil is varying due to natural and manmade causes that imbalance the input (addition) and output (depletion) ratio. The positive balance is essential for the soil fertility and crop productivity. The carbon source in the form of CO_2 absorbed from the atmosphere by floras in the soil and deposited as either organic or inorganic form in the soil particles for long period of time through natural process. The negative balance is being occurring in the soil when the uptake is more than addition. So, the basic understanding on factor responsible for carbon deposition and depletion is required to sustain the carbon load in soil ecosystem for its utilization by flora and fauna (**Table 2**).

5. Sources of carbon to the soil ecosystem

5.1 Soil organic matter cycling

The type of soil, climatic factors, and management practices influence the organic matter addition to soil through its turnover or decomposition. Among the weather factors, rainfall is critical for plant growth and soil microbial activity, which leads to decomposition of organic residues available in the soil ecosystem. There are different soil organic matter fractions, viz. particulate, dissolved, humus, and resistant types. Their turn over in the soil is very different in terms of duration (**Table 3**). Furthermore, soil organic matter cycles occurring continuously between livings, stable and decomposing fractions in the soil (**Figure 3**).

5.2 Natural carbon cycle

Carbon cycle is the combination of different processes like respiration, translocation, absorption, photosynthesis, and decomposition. In the carbon cycle, carbon containing living and nonliving things are cycling between different ecosystems, like terrestrial, aquatic, forest with living organisms in the atmosphere. The carbon element is taken up by plants from the atmosphere through respiration for food

S. No	Microorganisms	Function in the soil
1.	Bacteria	Decomposition of organic matters for nitrogen fixation and carbon accumulation Mineralization of nitrate and nitrite nitrogen and release of carbon compounds Oxidation of ion- and sulfur-containing organic matters
2.	Fungi	Decomposition of organic matters which releases organic carbon to the soil
3.	Actinomycetes	Absorption of nutrients and decomposition of organic mater
4.	Earthworm	Lifting of organic carbon to the upper layer of the soil

Table 1.
Microorganisms and its role in soil.

S. No.	Carbon status	Level
1.	Organic C is around 2 × greater C content than Earth's atmosphere[a]	60%
2.	Amount of carbon in top 1 m of Earth's soil [b] 2/3 as organic matter	2200 Gt
3.	Fraction of antecedent soil and vegetation carbon characteristically lost from agricultural land since 19th century[c]	25%
4.	Fraction of global land area degraded in past 25 years due to soil carbon loss[d]	1 mm $year^{-1}$
5.	Rate of soil loss due to conventional agriculture tillage soil formation[e]	0.01 mm $year^{-1}$
6.	Global mean land denudation rate [a, f]	0.06 mm $year^{-1}$
7.	Rate of peat lands loss due to drainage compared to peat accumulation rate[g]	20× faster
8.	Equivalent fraction of anthropogenic greenhouse gas emissions from peatland loss[g]	6% annually
9.	Soil greenhouse gas contributions to anthropogenic emissions, in CO_2 Equivalents[h]	25%

Source: Banwart et al. [8].
[a]*Rate of land lowering due to chemical and physical weathering losses.*
[b]*Batjes [9].*
[c]*Houghton [10].*
[d]*Bai et al. [11].*
[e]*Montgomery [12].*
[f]*Wilkinson and McElroy [13].*
[g]*Joosten [14].*
[h]*2004 data not including CH4, IPCC (2007).*

Table 2.
Fact sheet of global soil carbon reserves.

Microorganisms	Compounds	Composition	Amount in soil	Fractions for models
Nonliving organic matter	Dissolved organic matter	Litter	<0.1%	Labile soil carbon Active pool
	Particulate organic matter	Macro-organic material	5–20%	Decomposable plant materials (low C:N ratio, low lignin)
		Light fraction		Resistant plant material (high C:N ratio, high lignin)
	Humus	Non-humic biomolecules	65–80%	Resistant plant material (high C:N ratio, high lignin)
		Humic substances		
	Inert organic matter	Charcoal/char		
Living organic matter	Phytomass	Plant roots, litter	1%	Labile soil carbon
	Microbial biomass	Bacteria	2–5%	Active pool Decomposable plant materials (Low C:N ratio, low lignin)
	Faunal biomass	Fungal	<1%	Resistant plant material (High C:N ratio, high lignin) (High C:N ratio, high lignin)

Table 3.
Fractions of soil organic matter based on Baldock and Sjemstad [16] and use for soil carbon models [17].

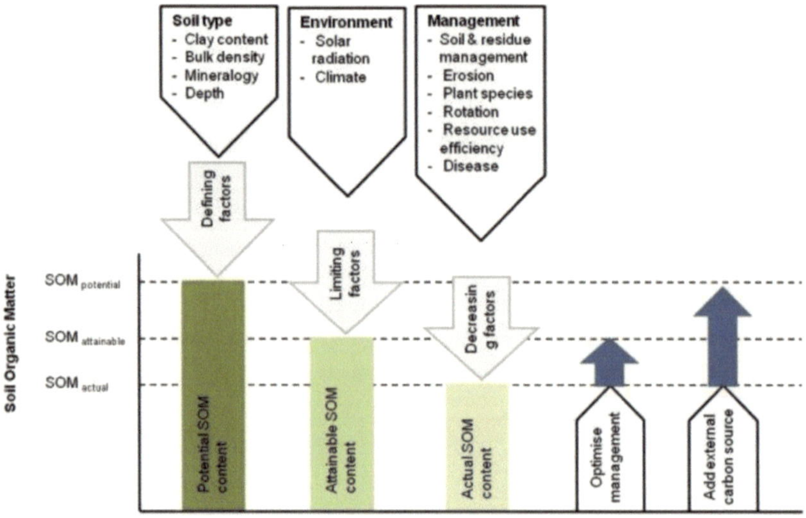

Figure 3.
The influence of soil type, climate, and management factors on the retention of soil organic matter in soils (Ingram et al. [15]).

production to maintain the food chain of the ecosystem. In the atmosphere, carbon is available in the gaseous form as carbon dioxide (CO_2) due to the attachment of carbon to oxygen. The carbon dioxide from the air is taken up by the plants to produce the food as carbohydrate in the presence of sun and water. Later, the carbon in plants and animals will enter into the soil ecosystem due to decaying process of plant parts and animal bodies after completing their life cycle at senescence stage. There are certain exceptional conditions like earthquake and tsunami, where the plant and animal parts will be buried in the deeper depth of the soil system which are converted into fossil fuel after millions and millions of years. The carbon moves from the ground to atmosphere due to burning of fossil fuels, debris of plant and animal origin. The movement of carbon from fossil fuels to the atmosphere is occurring in a fast manner due to burning of fossil field and then quantity of five and a half billion tons of carbon are released into the atmosphere (**Figure 4**).

Another important process in the carbon cycle is releasing carbon dioxide gas (CO_2) into the atmosphere by each exhale of living organisms. Animals and plants are getting carbon dioxide gas through the respiration process.

The role of carbon for regulation of global climate is inevitable. The activities of living organisms on the Earth, including the human beings, increased the carbon releasing form as carbon dioxide through burning of crop residues and fossil fuels. Forest ecosystem is a major sink for carbon. But, the deforestation due to infrastructure development and forest fire are causing the leaf mass reduction, which ultimately affect the CO_2 sink in the ecosystem. The floral green masses are major storage green cylinder for CO_2, especially during photosynthesis to produce carbohydrate (CHO). On the other hand, the atmospheric carbon concentration is an increasing trend due to population, urbanization, changing life styles, etc., which ultimately affect the climatic condition of the region, habitat loss, floral and faunal extinction, and health risk to human and animals due to global warming.

5.3 Decomposing of natural flora and fauna

The decomposition of plant and animal residues will result in the formation of different soil organic carbon fractions, which ultimately improves the pH buffering

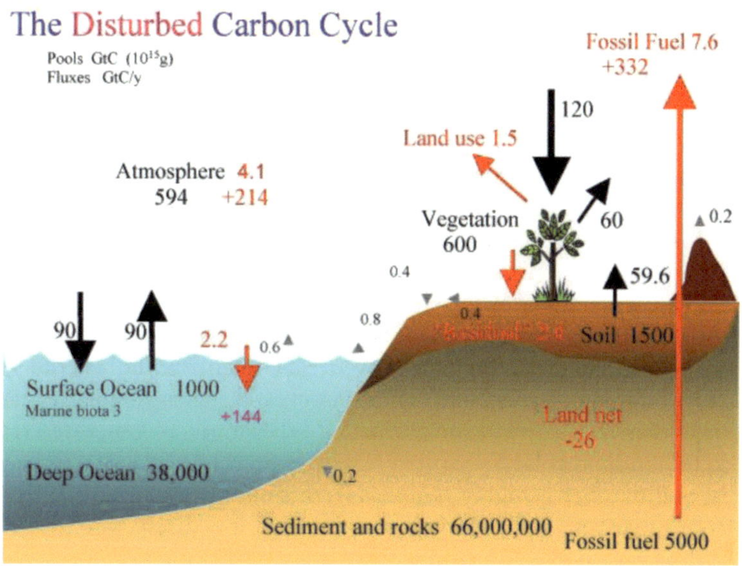

Figure 4.
Carbon cycle in between both natural and manmade fluxes. Ning Zeng, 2008.

capacity and cation exchange capacity in the soil. The transformation of nitrogen-based organic crop residues occurs during decomposition to inorganic molecules; for example, organic nitrogen (N) to ammonia ($NH4^{+}$) and nitrate ($NO_3^{\ -}$) adds nutrient to soil and also organic matter. Sometimes, the production of these gases (CO_2, N_2O, NH_3, N_2, and CH_4) contributes to the greenhouse effect and global warming. The beneficial microbial agents like bacteria, fungi, and actinomycetes are decompose the organic residues available on the soil and make around 90% of the organic carbon entering in soil. In doing so, they respire the carbon back into the atmosphere as carbon dioxide. Based on the soil types and climatic conditions, 30% of organic inputs are converted into humus due to activity of microorganisms. The clay soils will retain more organic matter than sandy soils, so the organic carbon content also increased. The cool climatic condition will not favor for the microbial action on organic residues which paves way for slow buildup of organic carbon in the soil.

5.4 Industrial organic wastes

The waste materials are generated by various industrial sectors in the different parts of the country. Organic wastes such as cassava rind, sugarcane bagasse, potato peel, coffee husk, and banana bark have been used as a substrate in solid-state fermentation using different microorganisms for the production of aromatic substances [18]. It is found that most of the aromatic compounds are industrially produced by microbial fermentation [20]. The wastes' by-products produced from food and agricultural industries are voluminous and rich in carbon-containing compounds such as carbohydrates, proteins, and other nutrients, which can be utilized as a substrate for the production of chemicals and enzymes by the solid-state fermentation technique [21]. In this technique, the nature of the solid substrate is a very important aspect. However, the solid substrate contains nutrients for microbial multiplication and renders physical support for the growth of microbial cells. Currently, there has been an increasing trend toward the recycling of agro-industrial waste including sugarcane press mud and bagasse. Pandey et al. [22]

reported various processes on sugarcane by-products for different purposes like paper production, power generation, the production of paper, and manure and alcohol based on fermentation.

6. Role of sugarcane by-products for soil fertility

6.1 Status of sugarcane by-products

India is highly dependent on agriculture, which is the main income source and employment generating sector for its development. Sugarcane is one of the important crops; crystal sugar is produced in commercial quantity. India is the second largest sugar producing country in the point of crystal sugar production. The sugarcane by-products like bagasse, molasses, and press mud are generated from this industry; so to handle this large quantity of waste products in a safe and eco-friendly disposal manner is highly required in this hour. Press mud is a by-product obtained from sugarcane syrup during processing. If it is discharged into environment without proper treatment, it causes soil and water pollution. In addition, the sugarcane by-products possess many plant nutrients and organic matter to enhance the soil physiochemical and biological properties [23]. Sugarcane is one of the commercial crops and cultivated across all the agro-climatic zones of the world [24, 25]. Choudhary et al. [26] stated that the areas of the crops are around 26.9 million hectares (M ha) and cover more than 110 countries with production of 1.91 billion tonnes (bt) [27]. Sugarcane is a cash crop as well as long-duration nutrient exhaustive crop [28]. Though many commercial crops are available in different parts of the country, sugarcane is the maximum cultivated crop due to its commercial valued commodities like crystal sugar and jaggery and its by-products, viz. trash press mud, bagasse, for organic manure usage, and alcohol from the molasses (**Table 4**).

6.2 Important soil amending nutrient rich sugarcane by-products

Brazil is the first largest sugar producing country and then India ranks second. In India, Maharashtra state is the first in sugar production. So, industries are producing huge volume of waste products which requires safe and eco-friendly management practices to obtain the organic manure for cropping land. The press mud contains higher amount of nutrients, so it has to be composted to be used as biomanure for different crops. Among the industries, sugarcane industries are generating various by-products, viz. trash, press mud, and bagasse of nutrient-rich organic nature. Hence, these by-products have to be processed effectively for

States	Press mud	Bagasse	Bagasse ash
Punjab	0.111	0.555	0.094
Haryana	0.160	0.801	0.136
Uttar Pradesh	3.516	17.571	2.987
Karnataka	0.913	4.566	0.773
Maharashtra	1.925	9.624	1.630
All India	**8.774**	**43.845**	**7.454**

Table 4.
Sugarcane by-products produced by the sugar mills in India (Mt) [29] (Fertilizer Statistics 2011).

utilizing as nutrient source for various crop cultivation programs and incorporated as reclaim the problem soil especially sodic soil.

7. Press mud

The estimated production of crystal sugar is around 354.95 million tons in the world and nearly 704 sugar mills are running in India. The sugarcane by-products are about 8 million tons in the form of press mud [30]. Press mud is used as biocompost to maintain the soil fertility and increase the crop productivity because the by-products contains the maximum amount of nutrients, viz. cellulose, hemicellulose, fiber, organic carbon in addition to nitrogen, phosphorus, potassium, magnesium, and calcium; and the micronutrients like zinc (Zn), iron (Fe), Copper (Cu), and manganese (Mn) [31] and also contains beneficial microorganisms. These by products are holding many beneficial effects on soil properties particularly the fertility, which ultimately increase the productivity of the crop [32].

The advantage of applying the organic inputs to the soil environment will prevent indiscriminate usage of chemical fertilizer to the soil. The composted press mud manure is produced after drying crop residues to maintain the moisture content and also for active microbial population [33].

The well-decomposed press mud is odorless, dark brown, soft, and spongy nature with many cellulosic and hemic cellulosic materials including fibers, wax, and organic aggregates [34]. The cost of chemical fertilizers is increasing in rapid manner which results unaffordable by cultivators, so the by-products like press mud has promise as a cheap cost source of plant nutrient for cost effective crop production and also for improvement in the physical parameters like texture, structure, porosity, water-holding capacity, and moisture content.

The chemical characteristics such as pH, electrical conductivity (EC), cation exchange capacity (CEC), and biological factors like microbial pollution have been improved due to application of composted press mud [35]. The by-products of sugar industry can be utilized for carbon sequestration, which means transferring of carbon fractions or CO_2 into various carbon pools like forest, soil for long periods of time that can be stored [36]. Application of press mud as an organic manure shows 150% increase in the organic carbon after first application, and it has the potential to store more carbon and also help in reducing the impact of global warming.

7.1 Nutrient status of the press mud

Sugarcane press mud contains many nutrients, so it can be applied as organic manure to the crop and composted for value addition for easy uptake by the plants. Generally, the compost sample contains C/N ratio of 725.95, total potassium of 1.43%, and total organic carbon of 12.53%. The organic residues inoculated with microbial cultures such as *Trichoderma*, *Aspergillus niger*, *Pleurotus*, and *Phanerochaete* are effectively reducing the wastes into valuable organic manure (**Table 5**). This final organic manure contains maximum amount of nutrients so it can directly be applied to the agriculture field to meet out the nutrient requirement of crops.

7.2 Effect of press mud on soil physical properties

Generally, the addition of organic residues to soil maximizes the organic carbon content and also activate the other nutrients [36]. Further, the application of organic compounds enhances the microbial population and microbial diversity in

Sl. No.	Parameter	Raw press mud	Unit
1	pH	6.25	
2	Electrical conductivity	6.554	mS/cm
3	Moisture content	72.50	%
4	Total organic carbon	12.53	%
5	Total Kjeldahl nitrogen	0.48	%
6	Total phosphorus (as P_2O_5)	0.40	%
7	Total potassium (as K_2O)	1.09	%
8	C/N ratio	25.95	
9	Iron	0.15	mg/kg

Table 5.
Nutrient composition of raw press mud from sugar industry.

the soil, because the organic residues contain organic sources for its energy [37]. The organic source like filter cake increased the cation exchange capacity for 30 months after its application [38], and the residual effect remains up to 4 years in soil [39]. Regular addition of organic materials such as press mud compost, municipal biosolids, animal manures, and crop residues is of most importance in maintaining the tilth, fertility, and productivity of agricultural soils [40]. Press mud or filter cake is one of the important organic by-products of sugar industry which is capable of supplying sufficient amount of plant nutrients to soil, due to its favorable effects on soil texture, structure, water holding capacity, infiltration, soil porosity, hydraulic properties, and bulk density of soil, and can be linked to most of the fundamental soil properties [41]. However, these are accompanied by improvements in soil aggregate stability [42]. The physical environments of the soil ecosystem are critical for a healthy soil and sustainable agriculture. The higher amount of N, P, and K in soil has made it a valuable nutrient resource, which is due to increased SOM by adding press mud compost [42]. Addition of press mud improves soil aeration and drainage in heavy soils, whereas in sandy soils, it helps in improving the retention of moisture. When added to agriculture fields, it increased the cane yield, improved the juice quality, and enhanced the ammonifying power of the soils [43].

7.3 Effect of press mud on soil chemical properties

Many research finding stated that the press mud can be utilized for crop cultivation and also to improve chemical properties of the soil. The press mud contains the maximum amount of organic matter and significant quantity of micronutrients such as zinc, copper, iron, and manganese. Therefore, the application of press mud will likely to improve the micronutrient status and enhance the beneficial microbial population in the soil system. Soil organic matter increases cation exchange capacity (CEC) through enhancing the adsorbing power of the soils and then producing cations such as, Mg^{2+}, $Ca2^{+}$, and K^{+} during the organic residues decomposition [43]. The composted press mud contains the essential plant nutrients such as nitrogen (N), phosphorus (P), and number of micronutrients in higher concentrations than soils [44] fertilizer value and have been used to replace or partially replace inorganic fertilizers to increase soil, available Phosphorus (P) [45] and exchangeable potassium (K) [46], calcium (Ca), and magnesium (Mg) [47]. Continued decomposition of more stable organic N sources as press mud compost over a sustained period regulates the subsequent mineralization of available N in soil [48], which is balanced by partial biological immobilization by soil microbes and this balance provide a residual source of N available for plant uptake. The CEC (capacity to retain and exchange cations) of soils is measured as the sum of exchangeable Ca, Mg, K, sodium (Na), and aluminum (Al) cations present per unit weight of soil; however, the level and balance of these ions are important factors in structural stability, nutrient availability, pH, and the soil reaction to fertilizers and other amendment [49]. The press mud contains potash and phosphorus, inoculation of potash mobilizing bacteria (*Frateuria aurantia*), and phosphate solubilizing bacteria in the composting materials that increases the availability of K_2O and P_2O5 in the wastes. This may be used later like other organic amendments.

7.4 Effect of press mud on soil biological properties

Soil organic carbon is a complex and heterogeneous mixture of materials. These materials vary in their physical size, chemical composition, and degree of interaction with soil minerals and extent of decomposition. An industrial waste like press mud is taken as fertilizer to increase organic carbon in soil, with an intention of utilizing the waste and building up organic carbon in the soil. Application of press mud greatly increased bacterial and fungal population in soil [50]. Enhancement of fungal, bacterial, and actinomycetes populations by the application of press mud in agricultural soils marks their roles in decomposition of organic materials to release nutrient for plants growth and development. Furthermore, the higher C biomass and N contents in the soils treated with press mud showed changes in soil organic matter content caused by microbial enzymatic activities. Application of press mud was responsible for a large increase in the number of non-spore-forming bacteria and various fungi including *Neurospora crassa*, *Trichoderma viride*, *Aspergillus* sp., and *Penicillium* sp. An increase in the spore-forming fungi, *Bacillus* and Actinomycetes has a positive influence on soil aggregate stability, which was observed during the final stage of composting of press mud [51].

8. Composting of press mud

The sugarcane by-products are not being utilized or underutilized due to less awareness. As per the views of many researchers, these by-products had the significant impact on soil quality when applied to agricultural soils as organic fertilizer. It improves the soil health and sustainable agronomic productivity. Press mud is a by-product of sugar industry and for every 100 tons of sugarcane crushed, about 3 tons of press mud cake is left behind as by-product. When this by-product is composted, it is converted into a very nutritive organic manure, because composting is a most promising technology of waste disposal, enabling recycling and solid treatment of waste organic matter and by this process, organic solid waste can be biodegraded and can be made suitable by composting and the final compost products could be used in agricultural fields as the fertilizing agent which is rich in micro- and macronutrients; with organic carbon or soil conditioner, it increases the microbial population, prepares beneficial microbial communities, improves microbiological standard and substance which can manage, store, convert, generate various important enzymes and thus, apply to the field without adversely affecting the transformation of organics and reduce odorous gas to release into environment so it is eco-friendly. It is also used to protect the plants from various soil-borne diseases and to maintain soil fertility and enhance sustainable crop production in the degraded lands due to continuous and excessive uses of chemical fertilizers and pesticides. The nutrient mixture act as a catalyst for accelerating the composting process and the microorganisms involved are

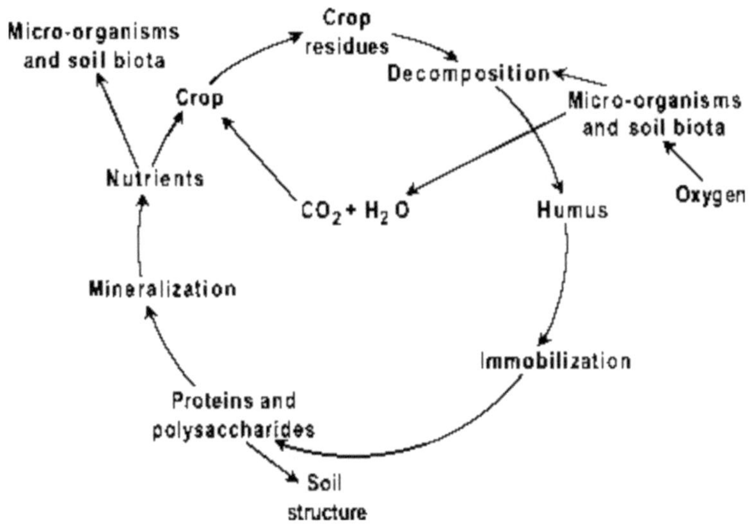

Figure 5.
Crop microbial decomposition cycle (Alexandra Bot, FAO, 2005).

Trichoderma, *Aspergillus niger*, *Pleurotus*, and *Phanerochaete*. *Trichoderma* is a fungus and also biofungicide, which is playing an important role to decompose the cellulosic matter of the organic residues into glucose. The fungus, *Pleurotus* is an Oyster Mushroom and a commonly cultivated species, and is also found in dead plants. The fungi are white or grayish brown or brown in color.

The important saprophytic fungus is *Phanerochaete*, called as white root fungus because it has the ability to decompose the polymers like lignin and chemicals at the moderate temperature of 40°C and efficiency changes based on the chemical content of the waste. The chemical composition of organic residues varies based on soil conditions, cane duration, cane varieties, and geographical variations. The crop decomposition cycles is shown in **Figure 5**.

9. Microbial biomass of press mud compost

The appropriate quality and quantity of organic residues are not only sources of organic matter and nutrients but improves the soil particle size, floral and faunal biodiversity, and microbial populations in soil [52]. The organic manure-added soil has maximum bacterial, fungal, and other microbial populations, which has a great effect on soil quality and sustainability [53]. The good quality press mud compost contain many nutrients and beneficial microorganisms (**Table 6**).

10. Sugarcane bagasse

Sugarcane bagasse is one of the major cellulosic agro-industrial by-products of Brazil and is being used almost entirely as fuel for the sugar industry. In recent years, there has been a tendency to use efficient agro-industrial waste such as sugarcane bagasse, not only as a fuel but also as a raw material for biotechnological processes, due to its lignocellulosic composition, which can be used for the metabolism of microorganisms to obtain products and metabolites of interest [54]. Sugarcane bagasse contains approximately 50% cellulose and 25% hemicelluloses and lignin. Chemically, bagasse contains about 50% of α-cellulose, 30% of pentosans, and 2.4% ash.

No.	Nutrients	Ave amount/100 g of press mud (%)
1	Organic compound	50
2	Calcium	11
3	Phosphorus	2–3
4	Potassium	1–2
5	Nitrogen	1.5–2.5
6	Magnesium	1
7	Sulfur	0.3
8	Cellulose	11.4
9	Hemicellulose	10.0
10	Lignin	9.3
11	Protein	15.5
12	Wax	8.4
13	Total bacterial count	3.6×10^8 cfu/g
14	Total fungal count	8.1×10^5 cfu/g
15	Total actinomycetes count	2.5×10^5 cfu/g
16	Total *Azotobacter* sp. count	1.2×10^4 cfu/g
17	Total phosphate solubilizers	2.1×10^4 cfu/g

Table 6.
Nutrients composition of composted sugarcane press mud.

A large number of microorganisms, including bacteria, yeasts, and filamentous fungi, have also been used in fermentation processes with sugarcane bagasse as support. Filamentous fungi, especially the basidiomycota, have been widely used and are preferred in the production of enzymes or enrichment of protein. The sugarcane bagasse contributes a significant proportion of the waste produced. In comparison with other agro-industrial residues, sugarcane bagasse is considered a rich solar energy reserve, due to its high growth rate (about 80 t/ha in comparison with 1, 2, and 20 t/ha of wheat, and other plants and trees, respectively) and annual regeneration capacity [55]. Another finding shown an increased amount of nitrogen and phosphorus due to application of vermicompost prepared with bagasse [56].

10.1 Nutritional value of sugarcane bagasse

The nutritional value of sugarcane bagasse is low when compared to other sugarcane by-products. It is highly lignocellulosic residues and contains cell constituents [57]. **Table 7** indicates the value of macronutrients of sugarcane bagasse for soil application.

Sugarcane bagasse	Composition (%)
Moisture	17.3 ± 0.35
Total sugars (in glucose)	30.9 ± 0.15
Protein	1.8 ± 0.33
Lipids	0.7 ± 0.15

Table 7.
Chemical composition of sugarcane bagasse.

10.2 Effect of sugarcane bagasse on soil properties

The average moisture content of the sugarcane bagasse was 17.3%. The filamentous fungi will proliferate well on sugarcane bagasse at moisture content of 50–70% to precede the natural decomposition [58]. The sugarcane bagasse having the moisture content of 17.3% means the bagasse has to saturate with a nutrient solution to increase the moisture percentage in order to grow the fungus. The lipids content was 0.7% [59].

Bonnarme et al. [60] reported that the low percentage of lipids in agro-industrial waste was not useful for the development of the microorganism. The carbohydrate is 30.9% of the wet weight of the press mud residue analyzed [61]. Another finding shown an increased amount of nitrogen and phosphorus through the application of vermicompost prepared with biogases [56]. Hossain et al. [59] stated that plant wastes can be applied as organic fertilizer and soil conditioner and used as soil amendment. El-Halim [62] stated that the water holding capacity attributed to the application of sugarcane bagasse in the soil is due to the coherent interaction of soil and bagasse particles cause soil aggregation. The soil aggregation property is responsible for soil water holding capacity. In [62], it is stated that the total sugar content is 16.4 % in unprocessed bagasse. Glucose can be used by the microbes during fermentation [63]. The filamentous fungus will grow rapidly in different substrates using different carbohydrate substances and produces different metabolites.

Carvalho et al. [64] stated that the amount of 2.0–2.4% of crude protein is found in the sugarcane bagasse. The crude protein content will be raised by the use of chemical additives like urea and ammonia anhydrous of non protein nitrogen compounds. Bagasse is explode as soil basel dose for the cultivation of crops which gives soil physical and economic responses in addition to productivity of the animals [65]. The overall facts on the importance of sugarcane bagasse management are related to disposal of agro-based waste products to the environment which causes environmental pollution [66].

10.3 Nutrient enrichment techniques like composting to enhance the organic carbon and nutrients of sugar factory by-products

The important organic by-product of sugar mills is press mud. This by-product is utilized widely as soil application to provide a nutrient-rich, high quality organic matter especially in subcontinental countries. The organic residue, i.e., press mud is dark brown material that contain macro- and micronutrients. The chemical compounds such as carbohydrate, protein, cellulose, lignin, and sugar fiber, which can be composited into carbon-rich final end product like biomanure [67]. The press mud also involves the production of biocompost and biofuel [68]. The application of pressmud at 20 tons per ha will save 25% of the recommended dose of fertilizers and also leaves the residual nutrient effects on the succeeding crops [69]. The press mud contains 25–30% of organic matter. Further, the pressmud contains major plant nutrients like nitrogen, phosphorus, potassium, calcium, magnesium, and sulfur in addition to the minor micronutrients such as Zn, Fe, Mn, B, Cu, Mo and also the beneficial microorganisms for the composting [70].

11. Composting process

The organic wastes are mainly used for producing organic manure through biocomposting and vermicomposting processes. The sugarcane by-products particularly the press mud is nutritive organic materials of converting itself into organic manure through proper composting technique. Generally, the composting of press mud will be carried out by inoculating inoculum of different microorganisms along with cow dung is an important at the initial stage of composting. The present study concentrates on effectiveness of various microorganisms on decomposition of press mud with a nutrient mixture. As per the literatures, four microorganisms are chosen for the study which is capable of decomposing the press mud as a stable material. Details of the same are discussed below.

12. Microbial compost mixture for sugarcane by-products

Based on many literatures, the general composting procedure is as follows. The collected press mud is dried to remove the moisture content. Later, 5 kg of press mud was weighed and added with 0.60 kg of decomposed cow dung followed by mixing with 2.5 liter of water. The microbial mixtures containing *Trichoderma*, *Aspergillus niger*, *Pleurotus*, and *Phanerochaete* were added to accelerate the composting process. The viable dosage of microorganisms for the composting of this organic waste was 1.0% of the weight of press mud. The mixture of microorganisms and wastes were mixed together to imitate the composting. Moisture content of the composting mixture was 40–60% for the growth and development of the microorganisms. The composting process in container requires proper aeration and maintain the optimum moisture and temperature.

Composting is major technique to reduce the volume of waste. It is a considered as the simple method for recycling the sugarcane by-products of the sugar factories to produce the nutrient-rich manure. It can be used for agricultural amendment to compensate the fertilizer dose in the fertilization schedule of crops [71]. Addition of organic residues to soils is an eco-friendly way to increase soil organic matter content and stability of micro and macro-soil aggregates. The effect of these organic wastes will vary based on the quality of the organic materials added to the soil. The effects of the organic materials on plant growth and the nutrient levels of the organic materials will vary from waste to waste and also one soil type to another. The reviews conducted by NSW Agriculture [72] also indicated the usage of organic waste for different crop cultivation.

13. Effect of sugarcane by-products on soil organic carbon

Razzaq [73] stated that application of sugarcane press mud continuously to the cultivating land for crop production results increased the considerable quantity soil organic carbon in within 5 to 6 years. The soil health has been increased because of addition of sulfur, carbon ions and organic matters. There were numerous findings on the application of press mud as basal dose in the soil for farming any crops like cereals, pulses, oilseeds, commercial crops, and ornamentals, resulting in increased crop productivity in addition to soil carbon build up. Therefore, the application of press mud in the land is a common cultural practice to improve the soil properties in many countries, especially the sugarcane countries like Brazil, India, Pakistan, and Sri Lanka [74]. Above all, the waste to wealth concept is highly suitable to sugarcane by-products because of its numerous traits to sustain the yield, improving the soil fertility and maintaining clean environment in and around the sugar factories in addition to preventing the global warming.

14. Challenges

The level of soil carbon in the soil ecosystem is under threat worldwide due to improper management of soil organic matter through the application of organic manures from crop residues, livestock wastes, industrial waste, etc. In the case of nutrient depletion, the soils are particularly facing the deletion of organic carbon for every cropping operation due to its utilization, and there is no recycling of crop residues in the soil. Instead, the crop residues are either burned or underutilized through heaping and landfilling.

The organic carbon in the soil is highly associated with soil structure. The weather factors like heavy rainfall will erode the top fertile layer of the soil. The cool condition will not support microbial action for composting of different organic residues in the soil, which ultimately affects the organic carbon content of the soil. The different soil management strategies are essential to recycle the carbon through management of soil, crop, and nutrient during the cropping programme. The zero tillage will reduce the physical disturbances to soil. The intensive cropping system should not be adopted even the soil is very fertile because depletion process of carbon is faster than accumulation. Adoption of integrated nutrient management through the application of farm yard manure and adoption of green and green leaf manures incorporation provides an opportunity for the soil to build up its organic carbon. To meet increasing chemical nutrient resource demands and maintain resilience in soil actions due to high-tech farming and climate change, we are in a position to recycle the waste products from different agro-based industries, especially intensive nutrient up taking by crop like sugarcane.

15. Conclusion

Soil carbon is the nuclear element for the fertility status of any type of soil which will be mainly associated with organic matter in the soil ecosystem. The content of soil carbon is very important to catalyze the soil to execute its functions like transformation of nutrient to plants, water holding capacity, floral and faunal biodiversity, and transformation of energy among the different species present in the food chain. The sugar mills are producing huge quantity of by-products like press mud and bagasse, which are heaped in and around the sugar mills resulting in an environmental pollution and health hazard to the human beings and animals. The way for the effective management of waste materials is a need of this hour because it contains many nutrients. The waste products can be used for crop cultivation as soil mulch, manure in the place of chemical fertilizers. The major problem in the disposal of press mud and bagasse is due to their bulkiness and difficulty in transportation. The effective way for reducing the volume of these materials is composting to utilize as organic manure to the soil to enrich its nutrient status. Further, the press mud and bagasse of the sugar industries will be used as an organic manure after the composting process, which is also nutrient for nursery plants, garden plants and different crops cultivated in main fields. Generally, the sugar industry waste products are slightly acidic in nature and contain higher amount of organic matter, so it will be highly suitable to reclaim the alkaline soil contain higher amount of sodium. The available nutrients in this waste materials are composted through effective and suitable environmental friendly technology to enhance its easy absorption by plant system. Above all, the waste materials have to be processed into nutrient-enriched organic products in a commercial mode for marketing and wide adoptability by different sectors like farming, industries, households etc., and to eliminate the environmental pollution.

Acknowledgements

The authors are thankful to IntechOpen, for their motivation to write this book chapter and patience in completing this task. We also thank Dr. M. Pandiyan, Dean, Agricultural College and Research Institute, Vazhavachanur, TNAU.

Conflict of interest

The authors acknowledge that we have not conflict with any findings and suggestions of other authors.

Author details

Anbalagan Krishnaveni*, Sivakumar Chinnasamy, Jamuna Elumalai and Pandiyan Muthaiyan*
Agricultural College and Research Institute, Tamil Nadu Agricultural University, Tamil Nadu, India

*Address all correspondence to: venikrishna25@yahoo.co.in and mpandiyan8@yahoo.co.in

References

[1] Shen SM, Hart PBS, Powlson DS, Jenkinson DS. The nitrogen cycle in the Broadbalk wheat experiment: 15N-labelled fertilizer residues in the soil and in the soil microbial biomass. Soil Biology and Biochemistry. 1989;**21**: 529-533

[2] Kay BD, Angers DA. Soil Structure. In: Sumner ME, editor. Handbook of Soil Science. Boca Raton USA: CRC Press; 1999

[3] Carter MR. Influence of reduced tillage systems on organic matter, microbial biomass, macroaggregate distribution and structural stability of the surface soil in a humid climate. Soil and Tillage Research. 1992;**23**:361-372

[4] Chaney K, Swift RS. The influence of organic matter on aggregate stability in some British soils. Journal of Soil Science. 1984;**35**:223-230

[5] Krull ES, Skjemstad JO, Baldock JA. Functions of Soil organic matter and the effect on soil properties. CSIRO Land and Water, PMB2, Glen Osmond SA 5064. GRDC Project No CSO 00029. Residue, Soil Organic Carbon and Crop Performance; 2004

[6] Baldock JA, Skjemstad JO. Soil organic carbon/soil organic matter. In: Peverill KI, Sparrow LA, Reuter DJ, editors. Soil Analysis - An Interpretation Manual. Australia: CSIRO Publishing Collingwood. p. 1999

[7] Drees LR, Hallmark CT. Inorganic carbon analysis. In: Lal R, editor. Encyclopedia of Soil Science. New York: Marcel Dekker; 2002

[8] Banwart S, Menon M, Bernasconi SM, Bloem J, Blum WEH, de Souza D, et al. Soil processes and functions across an international network of critical zone observatories: Introduction to experimental methods and initial results. Comptes Rendus Geo-Science. 2012;**344**:758-772

[9] Batjes NH. Total carbon and nitrogen in the soils of the world. European Journal of Soil Science. 1996;**47**:151-163

[10] Houghton RA. Changes in the storage of terrestrial carbon since 1850. In: Lal R, Kimble J, Levine E, Stewart BA, editors. Soils and Global Change. Boca Raton, Florida: Lewis Publishers; 1995

[11] Bai ZG, Dent DL, Olsson L, Schaepman ME. Proxy global assessment of land degradation. Soil Use and Management. 2008;**24**:223-234

[12] Montgomery DR. Soil erosion and Agricultural sustainability. Proceedings of the National Academy of Sciences USA. 2007;**104**:13268-13272

[13] Wilkinson BH, McElroy BJ. The impact of humans on continental erosion and sedimentation. Geological Society of America Bulletin. 2007;**119** (1–2):140-156

[14] Joosten H. The Global Peatland CO_2 Picture. Peatland Status and Drainage Associated Emissions in all Countries of the World. Ede, the Netherlands: Wetlands International; 2009

[15] Ingram JSI, Fernandes ECM. Managing carbon sequestration in soils: Concepts and terminology. Agriculture, Ecosystems & Environment. 2001;**871**: 111-117

[16] Baldock JA, Skjemstad JO. Soil Organic carbon /Soil organic matter. In: Peverill KI, Sparrow LA, Reuter DJ, editors. Soil Analysis - an Interpretation Manual. Australia: CSIRO Publishing Collingwood; 1999

[17] Six J, Jastrow JD. Organic matter turnover. In: Lal R, editor. Encyclopedia of Soil Science. New York: Marcel Dekker; 2002

[18] Soccol CR, Vandenberghe LPS. Overview of applied solid-state fermentation in Brazil. Biochemical Engineering Journal. 2003;**13**:205-218

[19] Macdonald AJ, Murphy DV, Mahieu N, Fillery Labile soil organic matter pools under a mixed grass/lucerne pasture and native bush in Western Australia Aust J Soil Res. **45**:333-343

[20] Hofsetz K, Silva MA. Brazilian sugarcane bagasse: Energy and non-energy consumption. Biomass and Bioenergy. 2012;**4, 6**:564-573

[21] Longo MA, Sanromán MA. Production of food aroma compounds: Microbial and enzymatic methodologies. Food Technology and Biotechnology. 2006;**44**(3):35-353

[22] Pandey A, Soccol CR, Nigam P, Soccol VT. Biotechnological potential of agro-industrial residues. I: Sugarcane bagasse. Bio/Technology. 2000;**74**: 69-80

[23] Jamil M, Qasim M, Zia MS. Utilization of press mud asvorganic amendment to improve physico-chemical characteristics of calcareous soil under two legume crops. Journal of the Chemical Society of Pakistan. 2008; **1**:145-150

[24] Tiwari RJ, Nema GK. Response of sugarcane (*Saccharum officinarum*) to direct and residual effect of press mud and nitrogen. Indian Journal of Agricultural Sciences. 1999;**69**:644-646

[25] Dotaniya ML, Datta SC. Impact of bagasse and press mud on availability and fixation capacity of phosphorus in an Inceptisol of North India. Sugar Technology. 2014;**16**(1):109-112

[26] Choudhary RL, Wakchaure GC, Minhas PS, Singh AK. Response of ratoon sugarcane to stubble shaving, off-barring, root pruning and band placement of basal fertilizers with a multipurpose drill machine. Sugar Technology. 2016;**19**:33-40. DOI: 10.1007/s12355-016-0438-x

[27] Factfish. http://www.factfish.com/statistic/sugarcane. 2016. [Accessed: 15 May 2015]

[28] Baldock J, Skjemstad J. Soil organic carbon/soil organic matter. In: Peverill KI, Sparrow LA, Reuter DJ, editors. Soil Analysis: An Interpretation Manual. Melbourne, Australia: CSIRO Publishing; 1999. pp. 159-170

[29] FAI. Fertilizer Statistics 2010–11. 56th ed. New Delhi: Fertilizer Association of India; 2011

[30] Sanjeeva Rayudu E, Srimurali M, Venkaiah K. A study on macronutrients of alkaline soils by using Pressmud. International Journal Scientific Research and Review. 2018;**7**:97-105

[31] Patil NN, Jadhav S, Ghorpade SS, Sharma AKB. Isolation and enrichment of sugar Pressmud (spm) adapted microorganism for production of biofertilizer by using sugar press mud. International Journal of Advanced Biotechnology and Research. 2018;**4**(1): 96-104

[32] Angers DA, Carter MR. Aggregation and organic matter storage in cool, humid agricultural soils. In: Carter MR, Stewart BA, editors. Structure and Organic Matter in Agricultural Soils. Boca Raton: CRC Press; 1996. pp. 193-211

[33] Arshad M, chaudhry AN, Shaheer G, Farroq S, Manzoor S, Raza A. Effect of Physico-chemical properties on decomposition rates and nutrients release during composting.

International Journal of Biosciences. 2017;**12**:330-337

[34] Mishra A, Khan MZ, Singh A. In-situ incorporation of Pressmud cake in sugarcane fields: Impact on manorial value of soil environment. International Journal of Engineering Research and Technology. 2014;**3**(2):2889-2892

[35] Nadoni NN, Ananth GS, Dhananjaya Swamy PS, Kerur MS. Performance appraisal of Co- operative and private sugar factory in Belgaum District–an economic. Global Journal of Management and Business Studies. 2013;**3**(10):1197-1204

[36] Dotaniya ML, Datta SC, Biswas DR, Meena HM, Kumar K. Production of oxalic acid as influenced by the application of organic residue and its effect on phosphorus uptake by wheat (*Triticum aestivum* L.) in an inceptisol of North India. National Academy Science Letters. 2013;**37**(5):401-405

[37] Singh S, Dubey A, Tiwari L, Verma AK. Microbial profile of stored jaggery: A traditional Indian sweetener. Sugar Technology. 2009;**11**:213-216

[38] Rodella AA, Silva LCFDA, Filho JO. Effect of filter cake application on sugarcane yields. Turrialba. 1990;**40**: 323-326

[39] Victoria R, Banwart SA, Black H, Ingram H, Joosten H, Milne E, et al. The benefits of soil carbon: Managing soils for multiple economic, societal and environmental benefits. In: UNEP Year Book 2012: Emerging Issues in our Global Environment. Nairobi: UNEP; 2012. pp. 19-33

[40] Parmer DK, Sharma V. Studies on long-term application of fertilizers and manure on yield of maize-wheat rotation and soil properties under rain-fed conditions in Western-Himalayas. Journal of the Indian Society of Soil Science. 2002;**50**(3):311-312

[41] Chan KY. Soil organic carbon and soil structure: Implications for the soil health of agro systems. In: Lines-Kelly R, editor. 'Soil Health. The Foundation of Sustainable Agriculture', Proceedings of Aworkshop on the Importance of Soil Health in Agriculture. NSW: Wollongbar Agricultural Institute; 2001. pp. 126-133

[42] Hussain N, Hassan G, Arshadullah M, Mujeeb F. Evaluation of amendments for the improvement of physical properties of sodic soil. International Journal of Agriculture and Biology. 2001;**3**:319-322

[43] Brady NC. The Nature and Properties of Soil. 13th ed. New York: Macmillan Publishing Co; 1990

[44] McConnell DB, Shiralipour A, Smith WH. Compost application improves soil properties. Biocycle. 1993; **34**:61-63

[45] Pinamonti F. Compost mulch effects on soil fertility, nutritional status and performance of grapevine. Nutrient Cycling in Agro Ecosystems. 1998;**51**: 239-248

[46] Pinamonti F. Compost mulch effects on soil fertility, nutritional status and performance of grapevine. Nutrient Cycling in Agro Ecosystems. 1998;**51**: 239-248

[47] Mays DA, Terman GL, Duggan JC. Municipal compost: Effects on crop yields and soil properties. Journal of Environmental Quality. 1973;**2**:89-92

[48] Gallardo-Lara F, Nogales R. Effect of the application of town refuses compost on the soil-plant system: A review. Biological Wastes. 1987;**19**:35-62

[49] Hazelton P, Murphy B. What Do all the Numbers Mean? A Guide for the Interpretation of Soil Test Results. Sydney: Department of Conservation and Land Management; 1992

[50] Ownen WL. International Sugar Journal. 1954;**56**:212-213

[51] Roth G. In: Proc. 45th Cong. South Africa Sus. Techriol. Assoc; 1971. pp. 142–148

[52] Kumar S, Meena RS. Influence of soil and air temperature on soil microbes under current climatic era. Agriculture for Sustainable Development. 2016;**3-4**: 102-111

[53] Sherwood S, Uphoff N. Soil health: Research, practice and policy for more regenerative agriculture. Applied Soil Ecology. 2000;**15**:85-97

[54] Pandey A, Soccol CR, Nigam P, Soccol VT. Biotechnological potential of agro-industrial residues. I: Sugarcane bagasse. Bio/Technology. 2000;**74**: 69-80

[55] Souza O, Santos IE. Aproveitamento do bagaço de cana-de-açúcar pelos ruminantes. Comun. Técnico: Ministério da Agricultura, Pecuária e Abastecimento; Russia; 2002

[56] Babaei AA, Goudarzi G, Neisi A, Ebrahimi Z, Alavi N. Vermicomposting of cow dung, kitchen waste and sewage sludge with bagasse using Eisenia Fetida. Journal of Advances in Environmental Health Research. 2016; **4**(2):88-94

[57] Souza O, Santos IE. Aproveitamento do bagaço de cana-de-açúcar pelos ruminantes. Comun. Técnico: Ministério da Agricultura, Pecuária e Abastecimento; Russia; 2002

[58] Sales-Campos C, Araujo LM, Minhoni MTA, Andrade MCN. Análise físico-química e composição nutricional da matéria-prima de substratos pré e pós cultivo de *Pleurotus ostreatus*. Interciencia. 2010;**35**(1):70-76

[59] Hossain Z, Fragstein P, Jurgen HA. Review on plant origin wastes as soil conditioner and organic fertilizer. American-Eurasian Journal of Agriculture and Environmental Science. 2016;**16**(7):1362-1371

[60] Bonnarme P, Djian A, Latrasse A, Feron G, Giniès C, Durand A, et al. Production of 6-pentyl-α-pyrone by *Trichoderma* sp. from vegetable oils. Journal of Biotechnology. 1997;**56**: 143-150

[61] Pereira RC, Evangelista AR, Muniz JA. Evaluation of sugar cane bagasse subjected to haying and ensiling. Ciênc. Agrotec. 2009;**33**(6): 1649-1654

[62] El-Halim AAA. Assessment of the potential of sugarcane bagasse to mitigate clay soil cracks using image processing technique. Egyptian Journal of Soil Science. 2016;**56**(4):561-572

[63] Mendoza DPG. Variações do secretoma de *Trichoderma harzianum* em resposta a diferentes fontes de carbono. Dissertação de Mestrado: Univ. Brasília; 2009

[64] Carvalho GGP, Cavali J, Fernandes FEP, Rosa LO, Olivindo CS, Porto MO, et al. Composição química e digestibilidade da matéria seca do bagaço de cana-de-açúcar tratado com óxido de cálcio. Arquivo Brasileiro de Medicina Veterinária e Zootecnia. 2009; **61**(6):1346-1352

[65] Mahala AG, Babiker SA, Gutbi NE. Improvement of digestibility of sugar cane bagasse by fermentation with chicken manure. Research Journal of Agriculture and Biological Sciences. 2007;**3**(2):115-118

[66] Vendruscolo F, Koch F, Pitol LO, Ninow JL. Produção de proteína unicelular a partir do bagaço de maçã utilizando fermentação em estado sólido. Revista Brasileira de Tecnologia Agroindustrial. 2007;**1**(1):53-57

[67] Kumar S, Meena RS, Jinger D, Jatav HS, Banjara T. Use of Pressmud compost for improving crop productivity and soil health. International Journal of Chemical Studies. 2017;**5**(2):384-389

[68] Arshad M, chaudhry AN, Shaheer G, Farroq S, Manzoor S, Raza A. Effect of Physico-chemical properties on decomposition rates and nutrients release during composting. International Journal of Biosciences. 2017;**12**:330-337

[69] Nadoni N, Ananth GS, Dhananjaya Swamy PS, Kerur MS. Performance appraisal of Co- operative and private sugar factory in Belgaum District–an economic. Global Journal of Management and Business Studies. 2013;**3**(10):1197-1204

[70] Soccol CR, Vandenberghe LPS. Overview of applied solid-state fermentation in Brazil. Biochemical Engineering Journal. 2003;**13**:205-218

[71] Haug RT. The Practical Handbook of Compost Engineering. Boca Raton: Lewis Publishers, FL; 1993

[72] Gibson TS, Chan KY, Sharma G, Shearman R. Soil Carbon Sequestration Utilising Recycled Organics - A review of the scientific literature. Project 00/01R-3.2.6A. The Organic Waste Recycling Unit, NSW Agriculture. Report prepared for Resource NSW; 2002. http://www.environment.nsw.gov.au/resources/warr/SPD_ORG_0208SoilCarbonSeq.pdf

[73] Razzaq A. Assessing sugarcane filter cake as crop utrients and soil health ameliorant. Pakistan Sugar Journal. 2001;**16**(3):15-17

[74] Ghulam S, Khan MJ, Usman K, Ullah S. Effect of different rates of press mud on plant growth and yield of lentil in calcareous soil. Sarhad Journal of Agriculture. 2012;**28**(2):249-252

Chapter 9

Review of Environmental and Public Health Impact of Automobile Wastes and Automobile Transportation in Nigeria

John Kanayochukwu Nduka, Henrietta Ijeoma Kelle, Emeka Chima Ogoko and Perpetua Chioma Okafor

Abstract

Automobiles are machines designed for transportation; it is a self-propelled vehicle with power source for its propulsion and is used for transporting. Most vehicles imported into Nigeria are rickety and are mostly out of use, and since there is no regulation with regard to quality and quantity of vehicles to be imported coupled with lack of technology to deal with automobile waste, large volumes of automobile waste dot the Nigerian landscape. Negative environmental and public health issues of automobile waste and automobile transportation result from the fact that its several components (metals, metalloids, polymers, etc.) on decomposition or expiration release toxic substances such as phenols (C_6H_5OH), benzene (C_6H_6), polycyclic aromatic hydrocarbons (PAHs), and so on into the environment, while on operation, automobiles are the most significant source of air pollution as unburnt diesel releases particulate matter ($PM_{2.5}$, PM_{10}), oxides of carbon, oxides of nitrogen, oxides of sulfur, volatile organic compounds (VOCs), smoke, soot and ash particles, metal oxides, as well as nitrate and sulfate groups. The aim of this work is to explore and draw out salient points from previous literature with regard to detrimental environmental and public health issues of automobile wastes and automobile transportation.

Keywords: automobile transportation, toxic chemical substances, environmental pollution, public health issues, imported auto-waste

1. Introduction

An automobile is a machine whose ultimate designed function is to transport men and goods. It is also called a motor car [1]. It is a self-propelled vehicle which contains the power source for its propulsion and is used for transporting passengers and goods on the ground, such as car, bus, trucks, articulated vehicles, etc. It is also a transportation equipment unit which consists of a frame supporting the body and certain power developing and transmitting units which are further supported by tires and wheels through springs and axles [2]. An automobile is simply anything vehicular that has its own power source and it is mobile. Eckermann, [3] ascertained that the first automobile, i.e., steam powered, was first built in 1769 by Nicolas-Joseph Cugnot, but the first powered gasoline was developed by Karl Benz in 1885 through manufacturing processes [4]. Most automobiles today are propelled by internal combustion engines. Tremendous growth has occurred in the automobile industry, after the designing of internal combustion engines. Today, the automobile industry plays a crucial role in the social, economic, and industrial growth of any country. Automobiles offer very advantageous help to man such as movement of people and goods to their places of interest (such as city to city, city to the hinter land, church or religious activities, markets, schools, tourist sites, cross borders of countries, etc.). Sports cars are for sporting activities, sometimes for other personal interest, luxury, and entertainment. Increasing the number of automobiles on any country road means increased traffic-related problem such as road congestion, increase in ambient air temperature due to engine heating and exhausts combustion, delayed time of movement, and traffic emission pollution. Gaseous pollutants from automobiles such as carbon (IV) oxide (CO_2), carbon monoxide (CO), methane (CH_4), sulfur (IV) oxide (SO_2), and nitrogen (IV) dioxide (NO_2) and particulate aerosols were reported in Nigeria above ambient level [5].

Another emerging problem associated with automobile transportation is the ever-increasing automobile waste, for the fact that large volumes of aging vehicles are imported into Nigeria, coupled with lack of adequate legislation on life span of vehicles to be imported into Nigeria. It become an all comers affair, and the effect is that aged, rickety, worn-out automobiles dot the Nigerian environment [6–8]. Climatic factors such as acidic rain, moisture (dew) and sun act on them as they corrode, degrade and decompose to release toxic chemicals into the environment. This in addition to others constitutes environmental and public health issue.

2. Classification of automobiles

Rajput [2] and Kirpal [9] classified automobiles based on the following factors:

2.1 On the basis of load

Automobiles can be classified based on the load or their capacity. The heavy transport vehicle (HTV) or heavy motor vehicle (HMV), which carries heavy materials, possesses large mass and is bigger in size. Examples are tractor, heavy-duty trucks, etc. They also have light transport vehicle (LTV) or light motor vehicle (LMV) which carries light things and is less in size (e.g., car).

2.2 On the basis of wheels

Automobiles could be two-wheeler vehicle (TWV) (e.g., scooter, motorcycle), three-wheeler vehicle (TWV) (e.g., auto rickshaw), four-wheeler vehicle (FWV) (e.g., car, jeep, trucks, busses, etc.), six-wheeler vehicle (SWV), and more depending on the carrier design.

2.3 On the basis of fuel used

In this category, we have petrol vehicles, diesel vehicle, electric vehicle, which use battery to drive (forklift, battery truck and electric car), steam vehicle (e.g., steam engine boat), and gas vehicle (i.e., vehicles that use liquefied petroleum gas and compressed natural gas).

DOI: http://dx.doi.org/10.5772/intechopen.88491

2.4 On the basis of purpose

They can be classified based on the purpose they serve, i.e., it could be passenger-designed vehicles, goods designed vehicles, and special-purpose vehicle (such as armored car, ambulance, etc.).

2.5 On the basis of transmission

Automobiles could be: (i) Conventional vehicles with manual transmission, whose gear ratios have to be changed manually while driving (e.g., car with five gears). (ii) Semiautomatic transmission system: Some automobiles are designed in such a way that facilitates manual gear ratios changing with a clutch pedal. (iii) Automatic transmission system: Automobiles with automatic transmission do not require gears to be changed manually, but they are capable of changing gear ratios automatically as they move.

2.6 On the basis of drive

They could be (i) left-hand drive (steering wheel fitted on the left hand), (ii) right-hand drive (steering wheel fitted on the right hand), and (iii) fluid drive (vehicles that employ torque converter (e.g., fluid flywheel)).

2.7 On the basis of suspension system

Automobiles can be classified based on the type of suspension system designed with it. We have three types of suspensions. They include:

i. The independent suspension—it allows the wheels to rise and fall on their own vertically without affecting the opposite wheels, e.g., swing axle, multi-link suspension, trailing arm, etc. [10].

ii. Dependent suspension—it has a beam (a simple cart axle) or driven axle that holds the wheels parallel to each other and perpendicular to the axle e.g., beam axle, De Dion axle [11].

iii. Semi-dependent system—in this case, the motion of one wheel does not affect the position of the other, but they are not rigidly attached to each other, e.g., a twist-beam rear suspension [12].

3. Components of an automobile

Since the seventeenth century, several attempts have been made to design and construct a practical operative automobile. To achieve the purpose of making a vehicle move, various constituents' materials combine to form an automobile. There are six major components of an automobile. They include the following:

3.1 The super structure or the body structure (frame)

This includes the chassis which supports the engine, wheels, body, braking system, steering, etc. It is the main mounting support for all components including the various parts of the body of a car. It deals with the static and dynamic loads without undue deflection or distortion [2]. Other parts of the body includes the bonnet (hood), bumper, cowl screen, deck lid, fender, header panel, radiator core support, grille, roof rack, rims and hubcap, spoiler, fuel tank door, trunk, door, door seal, door handle, door latch and hinge, door water shield, tire; central locking, window motor, window seal, windscreen, sunroof glass, fuel tank, horn, trunk accessory, and wing mirror and glass.

3.2 The transmission system

The main function of transmission system is to transfer power from engine to rear wheel via gearbox to obtain the various gear ratios [13]. The speed and torque of the wheels change in relation to the speed and torque of the engine due to the gears in the transmission. They include clutch assembly (clutch lining, clutch disk, clutch fork, clutch plate, clutch cable, clutch fan, clutch hose, clutch shaft, clutch spring and clutch pedal) [14], gear assembly (i.e., gear pump, gear ring, gear shift lever knob, gear couplings and gear box, which contains the idler gear, knuckle, master cylinder, bearings, counter or output shaft, pinion, and gear set), propeller or drive shaft, rear axle shaft, trans-axle housing, differential set (i.e., spider gears, differential seal, pinions, differential flange and differential clutch), speedometer, transmission set (i.e., transmission gear, transmission seal and transmission spring), flywheel ring gear [1], shift valve, speed reducer or governor and wheel and torque converter [9].

3.3 The internal engine system

This part of the automobile is designed as an engine. It is a device which converts chemical energy from fuel through combustion with air (inside a combustion chamber) into mechanical energy with the use of other components in the engine. The internal engine supplies the power which is delivered by the transmission system to the wheels through the clutch or fluid coupling [2]. The system is subdivided into three parts:

i. The engine components, which includes engine the block [15], engine shake damper, vibration absorber, fan belt, gudgeon pin, piston (i.e., piston pins, crank pin, piston pin brush, and piston ring), engine valve, harmonic balancer, accessory belt, petrol engine, camshaft assembly (i.e., camshaft bearing, camshaft fastener, camshaft locking plate, camshaft push rods, and camshaft phase variator), air duct, connecting rod (i.e., connecting rod bearings and bolt), crankshaft [9], crank case, crank pulley, crankshaft oil seal, distributor, drive belt, cylinder head (attached with cylinder head gasket and cylinder head cover parts), rocker arm, rocker arm cover, starter motor (starter pinions and rings), air blower, turbo charger and super charger, radiator parts (radiator, radiator gasket, radiator pressure cap, overflow tank, thermostat, radiator bolt), water tank parts (water tank, water pump, pump gasket, and water pipe), oil system (oil filter, oil pan, oil gasket, oil pipe, oil pump, and oil strainer) and valve springs and valve seal.

ii. The exhaust system, which includes exhaust pipe, muffler (or silencer), exhaust manifold and exhaust manifold gasket, heat shield, exhaust clamp and bracket, exhaust flange gasket, catalytic converter, resonator and spacer rings.

iii. The fuel system, which includes, air filter, carburetor, choke cable, fuel cap, fuel cell component, fuel distributor, fuel filter and fuel filter seal, fuel pump, fuel injector, fuel injector nozzle, fuel cooler, fuel pump and gasket, fuel pressure regulator, fuel rail, fuel intake manifold and gasket, fuel tank, throttle body and fuel water assembly [15].

3.4 The control system

It comprises of the suspension, steering, and brake systems. They are control arms or A-arms, shock absorber [16], axle, spindle, springs (air spring, leaf spring, parabolic spring, ball joint, rubber, and springs), tires [17], power steering assembly [18], steering arm, steering box, steering wheel, steering column assembly, steering shaft, steering rack (rack and pinion), kingpin, steering pump, strut, chamber arm, pan-hand rod, pit-man arm, stub axle, tie rod, tie bar, toe link, track rod, suspension link and bolt, idler arm, beam axle, swing axle, wheel alignment, trailing arm [19], automatic braking system, antilock braking system (ABS), brake fluid, brake lining, disk brake, drum brake, adjuster wheel, anchor, hydraulic fluid, hydraulic brake [20], inboard brake, vacuum brake booster, dual circuit brake system, metering and combination valves, wheel cylinder, wheel stud, brake roll, brake backing plate, brake rotor, brake lever (handle), brake piston, brake pump, brake shoe, brake hose, brake caliper pins and bracket and brake pad [21].

3.5 The auxiliaries

This part of an automobile consists of all the electrical and electronic components and battery system. They include audio/video devices (i.e., antenna assembly and cable, radio media player, video player, tuner, speaker), voltage regulator, alternator, gauges [22] (such as ammeter, odometer, manometer, hydrometer, oil pressure gauge, speedometer, water temperature gauge, pressure gauge, fuel gauge, vacuum gauge, tire pressure gauge, etc.), thermostat, ignition box, ignition coil, sparking cable, distributor cap, electronic timing controller, calibrator, remote lock, engine compartment, starting system (starter solenoid, door switch, ignition switch, switch cover, glow plug, and starter motor) [23], lightning (spotlight, interior light and lamps, headlight, fog light, trafficators, turn-signal control, license plate lamp and bulbs), sensors (air bag sensor, coolant temperature sensor, throttle position sensor, crankshaft and camshaft position sensor, fuel pressure sensor and automatic transmission speed sensor), navigation/GPS navigation device system, central locking system, battery system (battery box, battery cable, battery control system, battery plate and battery cap), sulfuric acid and distilled water [22].

3.6 Car interiors

Dash panels, secret compartment or trap, car seat, seat belt, seat cover, arm rest, bucket rest, head rest, carpet and floor materials, children and baby seat, and bench rest [24].

3.7 The miscellaneous and accessories components

These are minor accessories found in an automobile. They include air-condition system (air-conditioner clutch, compressor, hose, relay, valve, cooler, suction hose pipe, gas receiver, condenser filter, and cabin filters), bearings (i.e., grooved ball bearing, needle bearing, roller bearing, sleeve bearing, plain bearing, needle bearing, and wheel bearing), hose (fuel vapor hose, high-pressure hose, and radiator hose), adhesive tape and foil, air bag, speedometer cable, phone amount, rubber (extruded and molded), screw, nut (flange and hex nuts), fastener [25], split or cotter pin [26], rivet [25], draglink, dynamic seal, O-rings, shim, central console, glove compartment, washer, hood and trunk release cable and paint and sun visors [27].

4. Chemical constituents of some parts of an automobile

The automobile industry uses a tremendous number of materials to build cars, including iron, aluminum, plastics, steel, glass, rubber, petroleum products, copper, steel, etc. In all there are more than 6000 (>600) components of an automobile. These parts are used to create everything from the small parts such as dashboard needles and wiring to the big parts such as the engine block or the transmission gears. Due to the high demand of automobiles and technological advancement, suitable materials have been used for the production of automobile components that are durable and serve the purpose of the automobile. Some of the chemical components of the various automobile parts are tabulated below:

5. Environmental effect associated with automobile waste and automobile transportation

5.1 Menace of automobile workshops

Due to poverty and the dire need to own vehicles for ease of movement, these aging vehicles still attract customers from Nigeria's middle class and those at the lower rung of the economy [8]. Large numbers are taken to automobile workshop for repair and refurbishing. Automobile workshops are important considering public health issues because they are carried out in poor environmental settings coupled with lack of safety and hygienic lifestyle (eating with unwashed hand, wearing of dirty and contaminated workshop clothes for a long time, etc.) of workshop artisans, yet it is a beehive of activities because it has become the source of employment to several informal sector workers such as auto repair, servicing and refurbishing, auto parts scavenging, car wash, tire pumping and repair, auto-electrician, wheel balancing and alignment, oil sales and servicing, spare parts sales, water and food vendor, etc. [6–8]. Apart from esthetic pollution, automobile workshop contributes significantly to environmental and public health discourse. Several literatures have documented that pollutants such as heavy metals [41], benzene, nitrobenzene, gasoline fumes, exhaust gases, particulate matter, etc. are released by activities at auto workshops and automobile and have negatively affected surface and underground water and adjacent farmlands [42–44]. In major Nigerian cities, automobile workshops are in clusters along major roads comprising unregulated activities such as automechanics and panel beaters (car body work). Large expanse of would have been arable lands are occupied and polluted. Drainage system is blocked by waste generated from automobile workshops, heavy metals, waste oils, and noxious gases that are released into the environment, adjacent farmlands and food crops, which may possibly be contaminated by heavy metals and toxic substances. Exposed subjects at automobile workshops (auto technicians) are established to have high risk of cardiovascular and pulmonary diseases [45].

5.2 Automobile wastes

Importation into Nigeria of second hand ("Belgium") cars is second to none in Africa; therefore the Nigeria landscape is replete with many rickety and not road worthy, aging, and aged vehicles. Lack of spare parts and adequate technology makes repair and refurbishing of automobiles an uphill tax coupled with unfavorable weather condition such as high temperature (Nigeria been in the tropics), acidic rainfall and high relative humidity, acidic mist and aerosols [6, 7, 46, 47],

S/N	Major parts of automobile	Chemical component	References
1	Car body	Iron-carbon Al, Mg, silicon alloy, Al, Mg alloy	[28]
2	Chassis	Al, Mg, alloy	[29]
3	Bumper/trunk	Fiber glass composite or acrylonitrile butadiene styrene, steel Al	[29]
4	Door panel	Carbon, Fe, steel, or Al	[30]
5	Window shields	Consist of glass made from Kevlar (poly-parc phenylene terephthalamide), K_2O, MgO, Al_2O_3 Polymethylmethacrylate	[30]
6	Rims	Alloy wheel rims consisting of Al/Mg	[29]
7	Radiator cores and tanks	Alloy of Cu, Zn, and steel	[30]
8	Tires and tubes	Elastomers, oils, resins, carbon black, steel cord and silica, contains natural and synthetic rubber (styrene-butadiene rubber (SBR))	[30]
9	Wheels	Al, Mg, Si, Cu	[30]
10	Glass	SiO_2	[30]
11	Sun visor	Made from substrates of polypropylene	[31]
12	Racks	Al alloys	[32]
13	Rivets	Al alloys, steel, Cu, Fe, Ni	[33]
14	Batter, battery case, plates, and connectors	Ni, Cd, Pb, HDPE	[22]
15	Pumps and valves	Cu, Co, Be, Al	[30]
16	Automotive exhaust system components	Cr, Ni, Si, Fe, Mn	[2]
17	Engine block	C, Si, Mn, Fe, Ni, Zn, Cu, Mg	[29]
18	Engine bearings, bushings, valves	Fe, Cu, Sn, and Zn	[2]
19	Engine cylinder	Cast iron and Al alloy	[2]
20	Hubcap: also known as wheel cover	Plastics	[34]
21	Radiator	Aluminum sheets	[35]
22	Multi-suspension system	Forged from aluminum system	[32]
23	Cotter or spilt pin	Cr, Fe, Cu, Zn, Al, Mg	[36]
24	Axles	Cr/Mo	[30]
25	Tie rod, pinion, and steering column	Stainless steel and Al	[32, 34, 37]
26	Steering arms	C, Fe, and Cr	[38, 39]
27	Suspension coils and springs	Fe, Mn, Si, P, V, Ni, Cr, Sn, Zn, Al, and C	[30]
28	Clutch assembly	Cu, Sn, and P	[30]
29	Gear assembly system	Cu, Zn, and steel	[25, 30, 40]
30	Crankshafts	Mn, Cr, Mo, Ni, Si, Co, V, Al	[30]

Cd = cadmium, Fe = iron, C = carbon, Al = aluminum, Si = silicon, Mg = magnesium, Cu = copper, Zn = zinc, Co = cobalt, Be = beryllium, Ni = nickel, Cr = chromium, Mg = manganese, Sn = tin, Mo = molybdenum, V = vanadium, K_2O = potassium oxide, MgO = magnesium oxide, SiO_2 = silicon (IV) oxide. Alloy = a combination of two or more metals, steel = an alloy of iron and carbon, and HDPE = high-density polyethylene.

Table 1.
Some chemical component of automobile parts.

unequaled and unprecedented high level road accident occasioned by poor road infrastructure and network, the net effect is that many vehicles are out of use and ultimately become waste. Recently wastes are regarded as "materials out of place" as against previous concept of "objects of non-usefulness." Automobile wastes are sometimes regarded as bulky waste, which include waste generated from servicing vehicles, automobiles, motorized trucks, and related equipment; they are made up of waste battery, scrap metal, used motor oils and lubricants, hydraulic fluids, bottom sludge, old motor parts, greases, waste engine oil, paints, petrol and diesel, which are generated and disposed indiscriminately. Abandoned vehicles dot Nigerian environment (workshops, roads, institutions, homes etc.) where they are left to the vagaries of weather to decompose and release some toxic substances, documented in **Table 1**, into the environment (**Figures 1** and **2**).

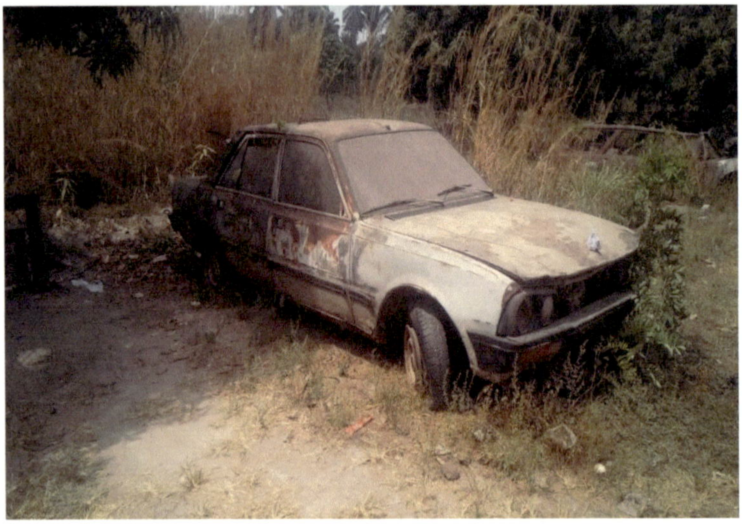

Figure 1.
Decomposing automobile wastes along Awka portion of Enugu-Onitsha Federal Highway.

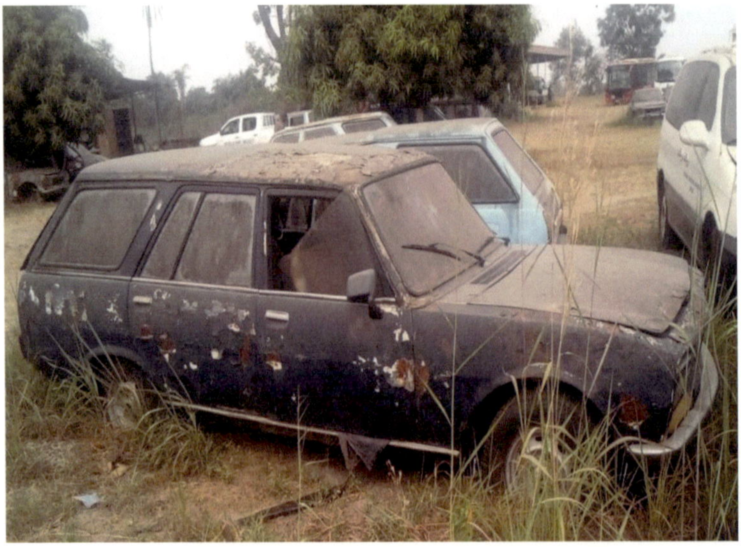

Figure 2.
Decomposing automobile wastes at Nnamdi Azikiwe university, Awka works department.

6. Greenhouse effect, global warming and acid rain

Greenhouse gases are gases that are capable of absorbing infrared radiation emitted from the earth's surface and reradiate them back to the earth surface.

The major component chemicals of greenhouse gases (GHGs) include hydrocarbons (HC), oxides of nitrogen (NO_x—NO, NO_2, N_2O_3, NO_3), oxides of carbon (CO_x—CO, CO_2), particulate matter, sulfur dioxide (SO_2), photochemical oxidants and water vapor (H_2O), ozone, and chlorofluorocarbon (CFCs) [48]. All these gases are in higher concentration released into the atmosphere by automobile emission and decomposing automobile waste irrespective of transportation mode [49]. Negative health effects associated with high concentrations of greenhouse gases already documented include asthma, respiratory distress, cancer, birth defects, low birth weight in children, genetic mutations and premature death [50, 51]. The resultant effect of higher concentration of greenhouse gases in the tropospheric region of the atmosphere is the increase in the air temperature. Anthropogenic activities destroying the ozone layer contributing to global warming stem from manmade compounds and chemicals with high global warming potentials (ozone layer destroyer) [52, 53]. Synergistic effect of global warming is much evidenced on melting of global ice stacks (glaciers), rise in sea level, and flooding of coastal regions. Three gaseous compounds (CO_2, SO_2, and NO_2) emitted by automobiles are of the compounds known as acid anhydride of which SO_2 and NO_2 are outstanding for they significantly contribute to acid rain. Exposure to ambient concentrations of CO can have resultant formation of carboxyhemoglobin together with inhaled particles, which increase blood viscosity, thereby hampering oxygen delivery to the tissues [54]. A direct effect of gaseous emission by automobiles is acidic precipitation which affects terrestrial and aquatic ecosystems with attendant public health implication as has been widely reported in Nigeria [46, 47, 55]. Depending on the soil in nature, acid rain affects the soil. Acidic precipitation dissolves organic matrix and mineral matter largely present in the soil, which are K^+, Ca^{2+}, Mg^{2+}, Na^+, and anions (HCO_3^-, SO_4^{2-}, Cl^-, CO_3^-); these replaces the hydrogen of the acid rain and make the soil acidic. The pH of surface water may not change much due to acid rain because of the counterbalancing effect of water chemistry. Apart from acidic precipitation caused by SO_2 and NO_2 emitted from automobiles, minor concentration of SO_2 in air causes respiratory tract problem, irritation, secretion of mucus, and death at increased level of 500 ppm. NO_2 causes lung tissue inflammation at (50–100 ppm) exposure levels, bronchitis fibrosa obliterans (150–200 ppm) exposure, death (550 ppm) exposure [56]. Skin cancers and lesion, stomach ulcers, ocular congestion or corneal problems, and epithelial cell or leukocyte damage are possible health challenges associated with exposure to acid rain [55, 57]. The above chronicled facts show that emission from automobile transportation can synergize change in climate (alteration between balance in incoming and outgoing radiation elements over a period of time in the atmosphere leading to differed quality of air over time) [58] and that climate change is intricately weaved to human health.

7. Public health issues associated with automobile waste and automobile transportation

For the fact that automobiles are the most important vital means of transportation owing to their ubiquitous nature, portability, flexibility, comfort, and affordable cost (when compared with trains, ships, and airplanes), more and more people all over the world are purchasing vehicles for their personal, office, and company use. Some families have as much as two, three, four, etc. depending on their purchasing power. In Nigeria, the Federal Road Safety Corps (FRSC) stated that there are more than seven [8] million vehicles on Nigeria road [59]. The automobiles are helpful to human population, and they can transport people and goods to places of need such as offices, markets, schools, sporting events, hospitals, leisure centers, etc. This is made possible by adequate road network interconnecting the cities and the rural communities. The inevitable effect is the numerous public health issues associated with automobile transportation. The use of premium motor spirit, diesel, paints, and other gaseous materials [45] has led to the increased pollution and negative health effect. Incomplete combustion of fuel due to lack of air, poor mixing of air with combustion gases, and low combustion temperature lead to particulate matter emission; the whole property is a function of operating condition of the engine, lubricant oil, fuel composition, and the gas filtering equipment [60]. Substances that can be emitted from automobile exhaust include CO, H_2, CO_2, H_2O, hydrocarbons (CH_n), volatile organic compound (VOCs), oxides of sulfur (SO_x), oxides of nitrogen (NO_x), particulate matter ($PM_{2.5}$ and PM_{10}), soot [61], and metals such as vanadium, lead, nickel, cadmium, potassium, sodium, phosphorus, lead, zinc, copper, manganese, iron, barium, etc. [60, 62]. Other possible constituents of automobile exhaust emission include benzenes, polycyclic aromatic hydrocarbons, etc. The list above is considered as the exhaust emission, while the evaporative emissions are the vapors of fuel which are released into the atmosphere unburnt. The car exhaust emission has a great deal of negative effect on the human health and the environment. Car exhaust pollutants cause coughing, breathing difficulties, eye irritation, and distress to the respiratory system (throat, lungs, and chest). Specifically, heavy metals such as lead cause an occupational potent widespread human and environmental toxicant produced by burning leaded fuel and can interferes with normal functioning of red blood cells, thus hampering important enzymes in the body, damages and shortens the lifespan of red blood cell and cause anemia. Serious exposure burden can cause renal dysfunction, fatigue, arthritis, birth defects, hallucination, psychosis, autism, etc. [63]. Severe exposures to cadmium cause tracheobronchitis, pneumonitis, pulmonary edema, contacting cadmium by inhaling of cadmium-laden smoke fast rack respiratory, kidney, liver and bone damage. The bone becomes tender (osteomalacia), depletion of mineral density (osteoporosis) which accentuate backbone and joint pain, thereby increasing the risk of fractures [64]. Irritation of the nose and throat, headaches, dizziness, body weakness, cough, chest pain, and chills are inflammatory symptoms. Cadmium and its compounds are also carcinogenic. Nickel, when in the body, can alter its chemical nature but cannot be destroyed, and its binding to form ligands and transportation throughout the body depicts nickel metabolism. Interference of nickel with zinc, manganese, magnesium, and calcium physiologically is regarded as its toxicity [65, 66]. Myocardial infarction, acute stroke, and burn injury are disease conditions linked with altered serum concentration and transport of nickel [67] inhaling automobile smoke laden with nickel can lead to high accumulation in the lungs, nasal septum, liver, and kidney [68]. Erythrocytes and leukocytes inhibited production, blood vessel damage, vomiting, irregular and abnormal heartbeat, which are caused by short-term exposure to reduced concentration of arsenic. Malfunctioning of cells, respiration, enzyme cell, and mitosis are caused by arsenic because it is a protoplasmic poison; the main effect is on the sulfhydryl group of cell [69]. Documented toxicological and health effect of manganese include decrease in semen quality [70] and Parkinsonism [71, 72]. For the fact that manganese is recognized to have different neuronal deficits such as learning disabilities, emotional liability, hallucination, compulsive behaviors, attention disorders, low fetal birth weight, and infant mortality [72–74], it is regarded as a potent toxin. The mucous membrane is the major target of inhaled hexavalent chromium or chromium-containing compounds, and then it synergizes asthmatic reaction, bronchial cancer, ulceration, and perforation of the nasal septum [75]. Although the human body for its physiological process requires copper in trace amount, increased exposure to copper through inhalation of automobile smokes/fumes will lead to copper toxicity such as early childhood liver cirrhosis (ECLC) and gastrointestinal symptoms [76]. The ubiquitous nature of polycyclic aromatic hydrocarbons emanates from natural processes such as forest fires, oxidation of biogenic precursors, unburnt petroleum products and other anthropogenic factors, which are released into the environment [77]. PAHs are hazardous chemicals that negatively impair human health [78, 79]. Accordingly, automobile transportation is a veritable source of PAHs in the environment being an anthropogenic pollutant, and the urban atmosphere is laden with PAHs originating from incomplete combustion of fuel in the transportation engine [80]. PAHs being highly lipophilic and insoluble in water persist in the environment (air, water, and land), and many of its compound are known carcinogenic, mutagenic, and teratogenic to organism [81].

Particulate matter ($PM_{2.5}$ and PM_{10}) are tiny suspended microscopic particles like dust, soot, ash, solid/liquid objects, gases, and aerosols that can originate from daily life activity. They can travel long distance in air been less dense than air. Those that originate from automobile/diesel engine exhaust may consist of complex mixture of organic molecules (conjugated and straight chain), incompletely burnt carbon, oxides of metals, acid anhydrides, and phosphate, nitrate, and sulfate group. The respiratory system is the major attack site of inhaled particulate matter. Penetration of inhaled airborne particles through the airways increases with the increasing reduction in particle size for those >0.5 μm [82]. The health effect from inhaled particulate matter may be affected by the site of deposition within the respiratory system. Deposited particles within the respiratory system are influenced by biological, physical, and chemical process which includes dissolution into body fluids with absorption by blood, migration into cells by phagocytosis, and movement with mucus and blood fluid [83]. Cancer, asthmatic allergies, inflammation, cardiovascular and respiratory disease, and mutagenic and teratogenic effects are health issues associated with particulate matter inhalation [84]. Bronchovascular disease has been reported among subjects exposed to welding aerosol [85]. Cancers of larynx, nasal cavities, and paranasal sinuses were established in subjects exposed to and inhaled chromate paints [86, 87]. Pollution keratoconjunctivitis (PKC) was reported among children in hydrocarbon processing in Niger Delta area of Nigeria [88]. Among automobiles, it is established that two-wheeled vehicles (motorcycles) emit more particulate matter into the ambient air than four-wheeled vehicles (cars) and therefore more polluting effect. This fact can be exacerbated in cities with high traffic gridlock (traffic congestion) as vehicular emission poses great threat to environmental and public health. The united nation (UN) 1998 report states that over 600 million people are exposed to hazardous effect of traffic-associated pollutants after 21 years; this figure must have increased.

8. Conclusion

High voluminous importation of aging and rickety automobiles with engines of questionable combustion efficiency, weak and deplorable road infrastructure, and high road accidents leading to automobile breakdown and favorable elements of weather (high temperature, acidic rain fall, dew, etc.), decomposition of automobiles, and release of toxic substances into the environment is inevitable, and this is coupled with toxic substances emitted by combustion of fuel/diesel during transportation. For the fact that Nigeria lacks adequate technology to deal with automobile waste, including recycling, there is a need to put in place, strengthen, and implement legislation regime so as to regulate the importation of automobiles into the country. Nigeria with a population of over 180 million people provides a large market for auto manufacturers. The government can negotiate with the manufacturers to establish a recycling plants, and this can remove large volume of auto-waste from the roads. The government can also assist the citizens to purchase new vehicles rather than fairly used ones through car loans. Adequate monitoring program by vehicle inspectorate officers to ensure road worthiness of vehicles. Tax incentives can be given to citizens who agree to limit car ownership to one. The government can also establish a comprehensive mass transportation network system that can convey large number of people on a daily basis. This can reduce the number of vehicles plying the road on a daily basis. Periodic air quality monitoring can be carried out to determine the levels of carbon (II) oxide, carbon (IV) oxide, oxides of nitrogen and sulfur, particulate matter, etc. in the air. Alternatively, non-fuel means of transportation such as beast of burden, bicycles, and trucks can be resuscitated and can lead to a significant reduction in number of vehicles on the road, meaning a decrease in pollution level and minimal health risk. The conclusion is that automobile waste and automobile transportation have some negative effect on the environment and public health.

Acknowledgements

The authors would like to thank the Federal Government of Nigeria, through its agency, the tertiary education trust fund (TETFund), for funding this research, covering 2016–2017 (merged) institutional-based research project (RP) intervention.

Author details

John Kanayochukwu Nduka[1*], Henrietta Ijeoma Kelle[2], Emeka Chima Ogoko[2] and Perpetua Chioma Okafor[3]

1 Environmental Chemistry and Toxicology Research Unit, Pure and Industrial Chemistry Department, Nnamdi Azikiwe University, Awka, Anambra, Nigeria

2 Department of Pure and Applied Science, Faculty of Sciences, National Open University, Abuja, Nigeria

3 Department of Natural Sciences, School of General Studies, Federal Polytechnic, Oko, Nigeria

*Address all correspondence to: johnnduka2000@yahoo.co.uk

References

[1] Ifediora GSA. Plant Machinery and Valuation. Enugu: Ezu Books Ltd; 2009. pp. 65-69

[2] Rajput RK. Automobile Engineering. 1st ed. New Delhi: Laxmi Publications (P), Ltd; 2007. pp. 1-57, 401-560

[3] Eckermann E. World History of Automobile. Portland, USA: Society of Automotive Engineers Press; 2001. pp. 14-304

[4] Georgano GN, Thorkil RA, editors. The New Encyclopedia of Motors, 1885 to the Present. Dutton: New York; 1982. p. 688

[5] Abam FI, Unachukwu GO. Vehicular emission and air quality standards in Nigeria. European Journal of Scientific Research. 2009;**34**(4):550-560

[6] Nduka JK, Amuka JO, Onwuka JC, Ndowelle NA, Orisakwe OE. Human health risk assessment of lead, manganese and copper from scrapped car paint dust from a automobile workshops in Nigeria. Environmental Science and Pollution Research. 2016;**23**(20):20341-20349

[7] Nduka JK, Amuka JO, Sale JF. Health risk assessment of environmental lead exposures through scrapped car paint dusts from fairly used car painting workshops in Nigeria. International Journal of Medical and Biological Frontier. 2015;**21**(2):163-187

[8] Nduka JK, Kelle IJ, Amuka JO. Health risk assessment of cadmium, chromium and nickel from car paint dust from used automobiles at auto-panel workshop in Nigeria. Toxicology Reports. 2019;**6**:449-456. DOI: 10.1016/j.toxrep. 2019.05.007

[9] Singh K. Automobile Engineering. 7th ed. Vol. 1 and 2. New Delhi: Standard Publishers; 1997. pp. 1-76

[10] McLellan D. Corvette from the Inside. Cambridge, MA: Bentley Publishers; 2002. pp. 86-87

[11] Setright LJK. De Dion Axle: The First Step to Independence in Ward, World of Automobiles. Vol. 5. London: Orbis; 1974. pp. 500-515

[12] Crolla D. Encyclopedia of Automotive Engineering. West Sussex, United Kingdom: John Wiley & Sons; 2015. p. 2003

[13] Bhanuse CG, Kawde VH, Nare AS, Patil NP, Zaware PK. Design, analysis and fabrication of automatic transmission system. International Journal of Engineering Science and Computing. 2017;**7**(5):11777

[14] Kaleem SS, Madhu S. Design of manual clutch control system. Journal of Chemical and Pharmaceutical Sciences. 2016;**5**:240-241

[15] Williams R. Understanding Automotive Electronics. 6th ed. Oxford, United Kingdom: Butterworth-Heinemann, Elsevier Science; 2003. pp. 8-22

[16] Hiller VAW. 60: Independent front suspension. In: Fundamentals of Motor Vehicle Technology. 4th ed. Calex, United Kingdom: Stanley Thornes; 1991. pp. 368-369

[17] Jazar RN. Vehicle Dynamics & Theory and Applications. Texas, USA: Springer; 2008. p. 455

[18] Schultz M. Steering: A century of progress. Popular Mechanics. 1985;**162**(5):59

[19] Cook ME. Revere the Gear, Good Landings Are More than the Ego-Boosters; they Are Kind to your Airplane's Landing Gear Flight Training.

Frederick, Maryland: Aircrafts Owners and Pilots Association; 2014

[20] Bhandri VB. Design of Machine Elements. London: Tata McGraw-Hill; 2010. p. 472

[21] Henderson B, Haynes JK. Disc brakes. In: The Haynes Automotive Brake Manual. North America: Haynes; 1994. pp. 1-20

[22] Hartmut A. Auto-Electric Basic Technology—Part 1. German: Namibian project. 1997. pp. 10-30

[23] Horst B. Bosch Automotive Handbook. 4th ed. Stuttgart: Robert Bosch GmbH; 1996. pp. 543-544

[24] Allen J. Jeep. MBI Publishing; 2004. p. 152

[25] Smith Z. Plastic Gears Are more Reliable when Engineers Account for Material Properties and Manufacturing Processes during Design. Motion System Design. 2000

[26] Welsh R. From Tinkering to Torquing: A Beginner's Guide to Tractors and Tools. USA: Voyageur Publishers, MBI Publishing Company; 2005. p. 141

[27] Forrester S. Upholstery Basics. USA: Lulu; 1991. pp. 112-113

[28] Orłowics AW, Mróz M, Tupaj M, Trytek A. Materials used in the automotive industry. Archives of Foundry Engineering. 2015;**15**(2):75-78

[29] Hirsch J. Automotive trends in aluminum-the European perspective. Materials Forum. 2004;**28**:17-21

[30] Kalpakjian S, Schmidt SR. Manufacturing Engineering and Technology. 5th ed. Chicago: Pearson Prentice Hall; 2006. pp. 156-210

[31] Park DW. How to Restore and Customize Auto Upholstery and Interiors. Minesota, USA: Motor books; 2005. p. 132

[32] Saini VK, Sunil KA, Shakya K, Mishra H. Design methodology of steering system for all terrain vehicles. International Research Journal of Engineering and Technology. 2017;**4**(5):460

[33] Gayle VM, Look DW, Waite JG. Monel. In: Metals in America's Historic Buildings: Uses and Preservation Treatments. USA: DIANE Publishing; 1992. pp. 39-41

[34] European Aluminium Association. The Aluminium Motive Manual: Applications—Chassis and Suspension—Steering System2011. pp. 3-22

[35] Nagar UT, Trivedi BM. Performance analysis and design of automobile radiator. International Journal of Advance Engineering and Research Development. 2017;**4**(11):921

[36] Soled J. Fasteners Handbooks. Chicago, USA: Reinhold Publication Corporation; 1957. p. 312

[37] Cheta D, Adityamasur AW, Aditya S. Selection, modification and analysis of steering mechanism for an all-terrain vehicle. International Journal on Theoretical and Applied Research in Mechanical Engineering. 2013;**2**(4):72

[38] Sharma PC, Aggarwaa AC. Machine Design. New Delhi: SK Kataria & Sons; 2005

[39] Singh N. Suspension system. International Journal of Advanced Engineering Research and Studies. 2013;**III**(I):115-122

[40] Sclater N. Gears: Devices, drives and mechanisms. In: Mechanisms and Mechanical Devices Sourcebook. 5th ed. New York: McGraw Hill; 2011. pp. 131-174

[41] Idugboe SO, Twawari-Fufeyin P, Midonu AA. Soil pollution in two auto—Mechanic villages in Benin City, Nigeria. IOSR Journal of Environmental Science, Toxicology and Food Technology. 2014;**8**(1):9-14

[42] Ilemobayo OK, Kolade I. Profile of heavy from automobile workshops in Akure Nigeria. Journal of Environmental Science and Technology. 2008;**1**:19-26

[43] Iwegbue CM. Metal fraction in soil profiles at automobile mechanic waste dumps around port, Harcourt. Waste Management Resources. 2007;**25**(6):585-593

[44] Nwachukwu MA, Feng H, Achilike O. Integrated studies for automobile waste management and environmentally friendly mechanic villages in the Imo River basin, Nigeria. African Journal of Environmental Science and Technology. 2010;**4**(4):234-249

[45] Junadu MK. Occupational health problems of motor vehicle mechanics, welders and painters in Nigeria. Royal Society of Health Journal. 1982;**102**(3):130-132

[46] Nduka JKC, Orisakwe OE, Ezenweke LO, Ezenwa TE, Chendo MW, Ezeabasili NA. Acid rain phenomenon in Niger delta region of Nigeria economy, biodiversity and public health concern. The Scientific World Journal. 2008;**8**:811-818

[47] Nduka JK, Orisakwe OE. Precipitation chemistry and occurrence of acid rain over oil—Producing Niger delta region of Nigeria. The Scientific World Journal. 2010;**10**:528-534

[48] Soneye AS. Concentrations of greenhouse gases (GHGs) around tank farms and petroleum tankers depots, Lagos, Nigeria. Journal of Geography and Regional Planning. 2012;**5**(41):108-114

[49] Chernyshev VV, Zakharenko AM, Ugay SM, Hein TT, Hai LH, Olasik SM, et al. Morphologic and chemical composition of particulate matter in buses exhaust. Toxicology Reports. 2019;**5**:224-230

[50] Tanimowo MO. Air pollution and respiratory health in African: A review. East African Medical Journal. 2000;**77**(2):5-71

[51] Berstein JA, Alexis N, Bacchus H, Bernstein IL, Fritz P, Horner E. The health effects of non-industrial indoor air pollution. The Journal of Allergy and Clinical Immunology. 2008;**121**(3):585-591

[52] Nwaichi EO, Uzazobona C. Estimation of the CO_2 level due to gas flaring in the Niger delta. Research Journal of Environmental Sciences. 2011;**5**(6):565-572

[53] Chevron. Climate Change; Our Action Plan on Climate Change. 2010. Available from: www.Chevron.com/climateChange/globaluses [Accessed: 12 June 2010]

[54] Maisonet M, Correa A, Misra D, Juakkola JJK. A review of the literature on the effects of ambients air pollution on fetal growth. Environmental Research. 2004;**95**:106-115

[55] Nduka JK, Okafor VN, Omoche IO. Impact of oil and gas activities on the acidity of rain and surface water of Niger delta Nigeria: An environmental and public health review. Journal of Environmental Protection. 2016;**7**:566-581

[56] Bhatia SC. Environmental Chemistry. New Delhi: BS Publishers and Distributors, PVT; 2010

[57] Jeffs DN. Acid rain and the Eye; Director Water Resources Branch, Ontario Ministry of Environment, Personal Communication. 1980

[58] Bond RG. Air Pollution. New York: New York Press; 1972

[59] Mbawike N. 7 Million Vehicles Operate on Nigeria Roads FRSC. Leadership Nigerian Muse. 2007. Available from: http://www.nigeriamuse.com

[60] Golokhvast KS, Chernyshev VV, Ugay SM. Car exhausts and human ecology (literature review). Human Ecology. 2016;**1**:9-14

[61] Wardoyo AYP, Juswono UP, Noor JAE. Varied dose exposures to ultrafine particles in motorcycle smoke cause kidney cell damages in male mice. Toxicology Reports. 2018;**5**:383-389

[62] Saarikoski S et al. Investigating the chemical species in submicrons particles emitted by city buses. Aerosol Science and Technology. 2017;**51**(3):317-329

[63] Jan AT, Azam M, Siddiqui K, Ali A, Inho C, Haq QMR. Heavy metals and human health: Mechanistic insight into toxicity and counter defense system of antioxidants. International Journal of Molecular Sciences. 2015;**16**:29592-29630

[64] Jarup L. Health effects of cadmium exposure, a review of the literature and a risk estimate. Scandinavian Journal of Work, Environment and Health. 1998;**24**:11-51

[65] Das KK, Das SN, Dhundasi SA. Nickel, its adverse health effects and oxidative stress. The Indian Journal of Medical Research. 2008;**128**:412-425

[66] Coogan TP, Latta DM, Snow ET, Costa M. Toxicity and carcinogenicity of nickel compounds. In: Mcclellan RO, editor. Critical Reviews in Toxicology. Vol. 19. Boca Raton, FL: CRC Press; 1989. pp. 341-384

[67] Agency for Toxic Substances and disease Registry (ATSDR). Toxicological Profile for Nickel. ATSDR/TP-88/19. Atlanta, GA, USA: ATSDR/US Public Health Service; 1988

[68] Andersen I, Svenes KB. Determination of nickel in lung specimens of thirty—Nine antopsied nickel workers. International Archives of Occupational and Environmental Health. 1989;**61**:289-295

[69] Mazumder G. Chronic arsenic toxicity and human health. The Indian Journal of Medical Research. 2008;**128**:436-447

[70] Meeker JD, Rossano MG, Protas B, Diamond MP, Puscheck E, Daly D, et al. Cadmium, lead and other metals in relation to semen quality: Human evidence for molyboenum as a male reproductive toxicant. Environmental Health Perspectives. 2008;**161**(11):1473-1479

[71] Aschner M, Erikson KM, Tjalkens RB. Manganese and its role in Parkinson disease: From transport to neuropathology. Neuromolecular Medicine. 2009;**11**(4):252-266

[72] Sahni V, Leger Y, Panaro L, Allen M, Giffin S, Fury D, et al. Case report: A metabolic disorder presenting as pediatric manganism. Environmental Health Perspectives. 2007;**115**:1776-1779

[73] Henn BC, Schnaas L, Etlinger AS, Schwartz J, Lamadrid-Figueroa H, Hermandez-Avillamm M, et al. Associations of early childhood manganese and lead coexposure with neuro-development. Environmental Health Perspectives. 2011;**120**:126-131

[74] Sprangler AH, Sprangler JG. Groundwater manganese and infant mortality rate by country in North Carolina: An ecological analysis. Ecosystem Health. 2009;**6**(4):596-600

[75] Langard S, Norseth T. Chromium. In: Frigberg L, Nordberg GF, Vouk VB, editors. Handbook on the Toxicology of Metals. 2nd ed. Amsterdan: Elsevier Science Publisher BV; 1986. pp. 185-210

[76] Pizzaro F, Olivares M, Gidi V, Araya M. The gastrointestinal tract and acute effects of copper in drinking water and beverages. Reviews on Environmental Health. 2001;**14**:231-238

[77] Mastral AM, Callen MS, Lopez JM, Merillo R, Garcia T, Navarro MV. Critical review on atmospheric pafts. Assessment of reported data in the Mediterranean basin. Fuel Processing Technology. 2003;**80**:183-193

[78] Orisakwe OE, Igweze ZN, Okolo KO, Udowelle NA. Human health hazards of polyaromatic hydrocarbons (PAHs) in Nigeria smokeless tobacco. Toxicology Reports. 2015;**2**:1019-1023

[79] Tongo I, Ogbeide O, Ezenionye I. Human health risk assessment of polycyclic aromatic hydrocarbons (PAHs) in smoked fish species from markets in southern Nigeria. Toxicology Reports. 2017;**4**:55-61

[80] Chernyshev VV, Zakharenko AM, Ugay SM, Hein TT, Hai LH, Kholodov AS, et al. Morphologic and chemical composition of particulate matter in motorcycle engine exhaust. Toxicology Reports. 2018;**5**:224-230

[81] Haritash AK, Kaushik CP. Biodegradation aspects of polycyclic aromatic hydrocarbons (PAHs): A review. Journal of Hazardous Materials. 2002;**169**(1-3):1-15

[82] Gormer P, Fabries J-F. Industrial aerosol measurement according to the new sampling conventions. Occupational Hygiene. 1996;**3**:361-376

[83] Raabe OJ. Respiratory exposure to air pollutants. In: Switch DL, Foster WM, editors. Air Pollutants and the Respiratory Tract. New York, NY: Marcel Dekker, Inc; 1999. ISBN 08247 95210

[84] Hung JL, Tsai SS, Chen PS, Yang HY, Liou SH, Wu TN, et al. Traffic air pollution and risk of death from breast cancer in Taiwan fine particulate matter ($PM_{2.5}$) as a proxy marker. Aerosol and Air Quality Research. 2012;**12**(2):275-282

[85] Komarova TA. X-ray changes in the lung at contemporary forms of occupational Broncho vascular diseases from exposure to welding aerosol: Candidate of Medical Science [thesis]. Moscow; 2009. p. 106 (in Russian)

[86] Alexander BH, Checkoway H, Wechsler L, et al. Lung cancer in chromatic-exposed aerospace workers. Journal of Occupational Medicine. 1996;**22**:520-526

[87] Brinton L, Blut WJ, Kecker JA, et al. A case—Control study of cancers of the nasal cavity and paranasal sinuses. American Journal of Epidemiology. 1984;**119**:896-906

[88] Asonye CC, Bello ER. The blight of pollution keratoconjunctivitis among children in oil—Producing industrial areas of Delta state Nigeria. Ecotoxicology and Environmental Safety. 2004;**59**:244-248